M000201720

Parkinson's Diva

A Woman's Guide to Parkinson's Disease

Maria L. De León, MD

Parkinson's Diva: A Woman's Guide to Parkinson's Disease
Copyright © 2015 Maria L. De León, MD
All Rights Reserved

This book or any portion thereof may not be reproduced without the express written permission of the publisher, except for the use of brief quotations in a book review and certain other noncommercial uses permitted by copyright law.

First edition 2015
Published in the USA by *thewordverve inc.* (**www.thewordverve.com**)

eBook: 978-1-941251-48-5
Paperback: 978-1-941251-49-2

Library of Congress Control Number: 2015944766

Parkinson's Diva: A Woman's Guide to Parkinson's Disease

A Book with Verve by *thewordverve inc.*

Cover artwork by Ros Webb
www.roswebbart.com

Cover and interior design by Robin Krauss
http://www.bookformatters.com

eBook formatting by Bob Houston
http://facebook.com/eBookFormatting

Dedication

This book is dedicated first and foremost to my God without whom I would not be here. Secondly, to my grandmother, whom I resemble most and who also suffered from Parkinson's disease and did it with such panache. I only hope to live life half as good as she did; to my loving husband; my precious daughter Victoria, who is the joy of my life; and the women of the DNC-De Leon Neurological Clinic, who are the epitome of courage. Even in the face of insurmountable odds they continue to persevere in their faith and spirit of hope, smiling until the bitter end, saying, "All is well!" I also dedicate this book to my friends and colleagues who are women healers in their own right, who lead by example. Their spirit gives me strength to carry on the good fight even when my body fails me, as it often does.

It is their hope which I want to infuse and impart to all who read this book. After all, it is HOPE which makes a dismal today bearable because of the promise of the brighter tomorrow. Life can come at you fast, but despite the curve balls along the way, I would not miss the rainbows nor a Plan B left behind as a gift from Parkinson's disease, because they are all an opportunity for new beginnings or a second chance, if you will, and neither should you.

Your journey begins now in finding your rainbows behind the storm known as Parkinson's disease.

Love you, Dad. Thank you for always believing in me!

Diva

Di • va / ˈdi-va / from It. diva "goddess, fine lady."
from L. diva "goddess,"
fem. of divus "divine (one)."
A lady of distinction and good taste.

Why a Parkinson's Diva?

It is tough being a woman and having Parkinson's . . . sometimes it makes me feel like I am an enchilada short of an enchilada platter!

Yet, I am a product of my sweet grandfather's unconditional love and upbringing, which has given me the strength to persevere. He was the love of my life and I his. He taught me two very important things in life: 1) the love for an almighty God, and 2) the love for the arts and sciences. From an early age, he raised me to understand that knowledge was the key to mastering the world, as long as I always looked and acted as a lady of distinction, ready for any occasion. I was always welcome to join him in his business world of wheeling and dealing . . . but not until I was properly dressed! Along with my first poetry and history books, he included a book on etiquette. So, he created the roots of the diva in me, and I carry on his lessons as best I can every day. Who would send a Glamour Shot picture of herself to a residency interview? Me! Who would buy a car without even having a driver's license? Me! Each time life throws me a curveball or a bunch of lemons, I not only make lemonade but a lemon pie, and depending on my whimsy, maybe I'll even throw in a margarita—just to show life who's boss.

To all the beautiful women with Parkinson's disease around the world: I pray this book provides guidance and encouragement on how to maintain control of your lives and let your inner divas sparkle.

Table of Contents

Preface

There are a lot of books on the subject of Parkinson's, but there are few dedicated to young onset Parkinson's disease (YOPD), and even fewer focusing on the subject of women issues in PD as a whole.

For years, we in medicine have been practicing and dispensing advice on therapies, treatment plans, and dictating prognoses for YOPD, based on studies that do not reflect the patient's makeup. Most Parkinson's studies reflect the experiences of predominantly white, male, and older patients . . . because up until recently, that was what the medical books showed as characteristic of a typical Parkinson's patient.

As a woman who just happens to have Parkinson's and as a neurologist, I know for a fact that man and women are NOT wired the same. So we should take into account both gender and hormone differences, including whether a woman is lactating or is pre- or postmenopausal, when dispensing medical advice and deciding which medical treatment suits the young female Parkinson's patient best.

The face of Parkinson's disease today is not the same as when I started my training in neurology, which was not that long ago. Less than twenty years ago, I encountered my first young Hispanic Parkinson's patient. She had just turned forty and already had been suffering from Parkinson's for at least fifteen years. At that time, I was young and naïve, and other than being sad and impressed by her disease and age of onset, I did not think to inquire about her social life struggles. How did her marriage and family life survive such a long and debilitating illness? Did she have trouble conceiving or difficulties during pregnancies? What other history could she share with me? This patient is special to me in so many ways, starting from the first time we met and going all the way through the journey of her being the first patient I ever supervised from beginning to end for a pallidotomy, including assisting in the operating room. A pallidotomy is a surgically induced brain lesion in the globus pallidus, performed prior to the advent of deep brain stimulation (DBS) to control involuntary muscle movements (dyskinesia). The memory of this patient stays with me all these years later, throughout my journey as a physician, and now as I write this book. Later, when I became a fellow at Baylor College of Medicine, under the tutelage of world-renowned movement disorders specialist, Dr. Joseph Jankovic, I encountered a second patient who came to us with Parkinson's, in her twenties, and in a pregnant state. None of us, including the medical experts with whom I'd trained and been practicing for over twenty years had ever witnessed this unprecedented event. Most of us were at a loss as to how to treat her because the potential for harming the fetus with the treatment options back then was not known.

Slowly, over the years, I have seen a rise in the number of young women developing Parkinson's; however, it was not until I retired from practice—due to an ironic twist of fate in which I was diagnosed with Parkinson's and became involved in advocacy work—did I encounter numerous women in their twenties with Parkinson's. Not only did they have the disease, but many had given birth successfully, although their symptoms were exacerbated during their pregnancy, which was in line with the few studies available to date. Nevertheless, at the present time, Nebraska is the only state in the country with a Parkinson's pregnancy registry, so the long-term effects of the fetuses being born to mothers with PD still remain a scientific mystery.

Because so little is known in regard to women's issues in PD, a lot of the information and discussion presented here is still controversial and poorly understood in the context of PD. Therefore, some of the speculations and opinions are strictly my own and intended only to rouse new possibilities for trains of thought, potentially leading to new paths of understanding and knowledge to bring forth new and better treatments, along with further development within the field of Parkinson's research and women's issues.

My goal is to encourage a holistic approach to the female patient with Parkinson's. This cannot be accomplished without education, advocacy, and research—hence, this book, to provide a ray of sunshine and hope to those in the trenches living with the illness on a daily basis.

Given the lack of medical knowledge and research in the areas of gender differences in Parkinson's, I saw merit in writing about my own personal experiences, including my observations as a neurologist (specializing in Parkinson's), as a caregiver, and as a Parkinson's patient. I wish to emphasize the salient points of navigating the world of PD as a woman, in hopes of guiding other women on this journey, to help them become empowered with fellowship and knowledge, and to encourage female participation in the research that will ultimately affect our overall quality of life and wellbeing. For years, there has been a gender bias in biomedicine, leading physicians to preferentially not only test drugs in male patients but also study diseases in men.[1] This practice has not only put all women at risk but for years has limited our scope of knowledge.

For a moment, I wish to focus solely on the issues of gender. We all know that women have two X chromosomes while men carry an X and Y chromosome each. Although we share half of the genes, the apparently similar chromosomes produce the same proteins in and around the brain at varying rates depending on gender.[2] These discrepancies alone are enough to influence how a woman with PD might differ from a man with PD of the same age, ethnic, and cultural background.

For instance, women taking antidepressants and antipsychotics are more likely to have higher drug concentrations in their blood compared to their male counterparts. Women are also more likely (more severely and more often) than men to experience adverse drug reactions. Eight out of ten prescription drugs filled from the US market from 1997 to 2001 caused more side effects in women.[3] Women tend to feel effects of certain pain medicines more profoundly and become intoxicated faster than men.[4]

I know a bit about this, as I have treated many female patients, including my grandmother, and they as a whole (group) tended to have not only more side effects but more severe ones to medications of similar dosages prescribed to men. This makes treatments in women, even when they had early-stage disease, much more challenging. I personally had to undergo numerous trials of various medications, which eventually had to be stopped, switched, or in some way modified due to side effects. This was a great problem for me, as it is for any active woman who is trying to only make the best of her diagnosis and get on with her life. I was in a unique position because of my knowledge and training, yet it was still an eye opener to realize that medications which I had used for years and knew to be safe and effective with minimal side effects in most PD patients, particularly men, were extremely troublesome to me. I was either completely knocked out, nauseated and throwing up, or dizzy to the point of passing out! Not a way to live life, for certain, and I wondered how my patients had managed all these years. I also recall a few women who always seemed to not be doing well, despite an outward appearance suggesting the contrary. Perhaps this newfound knowledge will give insight to those continuing to treat PD, especially women.

Even though I was familiar with most of the tricks to improve or counteract the side effects of my medications, the entire experience was overwhelming even for an expert such as myself. For a time, it seemed that the side effects were worse than the disease, and I questioned whether this was a path I wanted to pursue. However, knowing that early treatment does make a difference in the long run, I chose to persevere until the right dose and combination medicine was achieved. This is what any physician would recommend, because not everyone responds the same; a little trial and error is oftentimes necessary to achieve maximum results.

A personal anecdote here: One day early in my treatment, I went for my usual massage to help with severe pain due to my dystonia. I was already feeling quite foggy-headed due to my medicines. After I was finished with the massage, my therapist stepped out of the room so I could get dressed, which I accomplished expeditiously, then exited the room rather hastily making my way to the bathroom. As I was walking toward the ladies room, I felt a chill, which I promptly ignored; after all it was winter and extremely cold outside. As I passed through the corridor, I noticed all eyes were on me, which I ignored and continued to the bathroom. I did wonder briefly why everyone seemed so fascinated by me today. Upon entering the bathroom, I realized the reason. I had forgotten to put on my blouse! I was parading about wearing only my lacy red bra and leather jacket, which happened to be wide open.

Despite all the dissimilarities between men and women with PD, women are not properly represented in scientific studies to address our needs. I hope this serves as a stepping stone to encourage patients and scientists alike to begin to widen the scope of scientific knowledge within the field of neurology and, in particular, within the area of Parkinson's disease concerning women's issues.

Furthermore, via this missive, I would like to remind PD women of all ages that they are indeed sexy, attractive, and radiant, and to give them courage to show Parkinson's who is boss—despite having a neurologic disease that is referred to by many as a "Public Disease." (Thus coined due to the notable Parkinson's symptoms, such as rest tremors or gait impediments, which patients cannot really hide or dismiss any more than a peacock can hide its feathers. *Look at me! I am different!*) Yet, these outward manifestations of an inner disease are what makes us unique. Having Parkinson's permits us to display our hidden artistic talents just as a beautiful peacock displays its own plumage with pride and confidence for the world to marvel at. Sometimes the courage we possess as women and people with PD can be seen through a simple act, like putting on a favorite shade of lipstick or a favorite pair of running shoes or even wearing a colorful hat. For me, a nice shade of red lipstick helps me face the day's adventures, gives me that extra lift and motivation to dive into what is the roller coaster world of living with Parkinson's disease . . . as a mom, woman, daughter, wife, healthcare provider, and whatever other hats I may wear on any given day!

My mission would be complete if women with Parkinson's around the world become empowered, instead of paralyzed or panicked by the disease, through education, self-awareness, faith, and a desire to be a better advocate for themselves and others. I wish to help you discover the joy of life after Parkinson's diagnosis. This life can still be full and meaningful even with its perils and challenges. So, armed with faith, valor, hope, and knowledge—and a handful of dopamine, along with some dark chocolate for good measure—we can still be wives, mothers, sisters, friends, lovers, daughters, caregivers, grandmothers, and professionals . . . anything we want to be. We are free to pursue our dreams wherever these may take us.

"God did not promise days without pain; love without sorrow; or sun without rain. But He did promise Strength for the day, comfort for the tears, and a light for the way."

~Author unknown

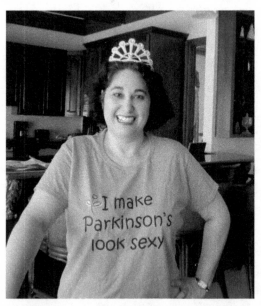

Maria in her Parkinson's Diva-wear.

Shirt designed by Alicia Friday
http://friday.wordans.com.au/T-shirt/i-make-parkinsons-look-sexy-618738

Livin' La Diva Loca

In my shoes, sometimes I want to cry.
In my shoes, sometimes the battles are tough to bear and the
*   scars are deep.*
In my shoes, sometimes life is just unfair.
In my shoes, sometimes the road is all uphill.
In my shoes, sometimes I feel is not worth showing up and
*   want to just give up.*
But tho' I often fall, cry, and struggle up the hill,
I always find a way to get up when I wear my favorite pair of
*   shoes,*
For in my shoes, God is ALWAYS fair and never gives up on
*   me.*
His strength in my shoes makes my journey with Parkin-
*   son's more than just a bear!*

INTRODUCTION

Facts & Demographics About Women

"Sex matters."
~ Lesley Stahl

According to the Administration on Aging of the Department of Health and Human Services, by the year 2030 the elderly population is expected to reach about 72 million (less than 19% of entire US population). It is estimated that if you reach age sixty-five, you will most likely live another twenty years. In this aging population, women are in excess of men by six million. Yet, 72% of men are married while only 42% of women are (a large portion live alone).[1] Half a million of these elderly have or will have primary custody of grandchildren. From other chronic progressive neurodegenerative illnesses, like Alzheimer's dementia, we see a pattern where women are typically the main caregivers even when they are ill themselves. We are now living in what is known as the "sandwich" generation, having to care for children while also caring for an older infirm parent, relative, or loved one. I am a prime example of this. At this time, even though I am the one with the chronic illness and stopped working because of it, my job responsibilities in and out of the home do not end. I still have to care for my daughter, husband, and my aging parents-in-law.

To make matters worse, at present most of the older generation lives off their Social Security benefits (87%), but even these limited resources may not be there for people like us who have YOPD. The future may be more challenging than we anticipate. Therefore, we must be prepared and make provisions for our future, especially since women are outliving men, and Hispanic women in particular are at the top of this list but at the bottom for resources. Other sources of income may include assets (52%), private pension (28%), government employee pension (13%), and earnings (25%).[2] These figures may be substantially lower, however, if a person develops YOPD and is forced to leave the work force early and, therefore, will not accumulate enough time or points in the work force to get a significant reimbursement from Social Security. This problem is not unique to our country; it appears to be the trend in various countries around the globe, from our neighbors to the north in Canada, to our friends down under in Australia, as well as the UK and Japan. Not only is the elderly population growing in leaps and bounds, in some places exceeding the working force, but the number of women doubles and triples in some countries compared to their male counterparts.[3, 4, 5]

The burden on some women as caregivers and providers is ever increasing as they too develop chronic illnesses at a young age, forced not only to leave a lucrative career or the work force completely. One national study on women and caregiving found that demands of caring for another person forced them to pass on a job promotion, training, or assignment in about 29% of the cases.[6] Other times, women may find themselves in an unexpected financial situation (a strained one) if their spouses are suddenly unwilling or unable to care for them and opt for divorce. In other chronic diseases affecting the nervous system, like multiple sclerosis, there have been studies, which indicate an increased rate of divorce. Although I am not currently aware of such a study among Parkinson's sufferers, from my personal experience and observations, I would say that the same holds true for Parkinson's patients. Women in general seem to be much more willing to play a caregiver role than are men. Women who are informal caregivers, in this country, are believed to comprise an astounding 59% to 75% of the population.[7] Therefore, when a woman, especially a young woman, suddenly takes ill with a chronic, progressive, debilitating, neurodegenerative disease, for which there is no cure, most men simply state they are ill equipped to handle this life challenge, some reiterating "they did not sign up for this," and so they simply bow out. This has been my personal experience within the confines of my own practice and within many of the PD support groups I have been part of. The burden then becomes not only one of personal health and overcoming disease, but a much bigger financial problem threatening the very existence and future happiness of those individuals, especially if they have no established support groups. Compounding this ever-present financial burden, whether married or single, is the ever-increasing cost of medications and healthcare, especially in the context of a chronic progressive disease.

The financial burden women experience is further heightened by the fact that women have typically been paid less than men for the same job with the same credentials and education. In the 2008 demographic evaluation of the elderly, it was discovered that even among the elderly, males made twice as much as women. (Median income for males was $25,503 in 2008 and $14,559 for women). So, frequently, PD women find themselves alone (with children) with a chronic disease and ill prepared for the challenges. Oftentimes, women with PD experience significant loss of wages and even loss of employment due to depression. This common scenario, unfortunately, only leads to a greater decline in quality of life over time, as well as overall decrease in financial stability.[8] A study referenced in Science News (November 2014) finds that "mental health issues lead people with Parkinson's to leave the workforce."[9]

Not only do women respond differently to treatment and present differently than our male counterparts, we also have more of our own unique stressors placed upon us by society than men do. Even if women are educated professionals, as am I, we are still obligated, or at least feel like we are obligated, to be the ones in charge of the family, the home, the children, the parents, the chores . . . the list goes on and on *ad infinitum*. We are good at multitasking, but what happens when we are the ones who get suddenly sick? Do our obligations suddenly banish or do they intensify? How do we cope, particularly in light of the fact that our risk of developing Parkinson's disease increases with age, just as our resources are diminishing along with access to healthcare? Hopefully this book will serve as a guide to help answer some of those major life questions as we navigate the uncertain terrain of living with Parkinson's and will provide a framework to set in motion plans, new ideas, and treatments that will benefit us all in the future as we age and deal with chronic illness, either in ourselves or in our loved ones.

1

Parkinson's Women Improperly Represented in Clinical Studies

"Be the change you wish to see in the world."
~ Gandhi

For years, women have been left out of the circle of new scientific discoveries and forced to accept the same medical guidelines for many diseases standardized with men in mind. One thing I have learned in my nearly half century of life is that if we want to make a difference, it has to begin with each one of us. A small ripple can have lasting effects long after the initial incident has subsided. We must be the first to value what we want to be valued, change what we want to change, and do what needs to be done. We must take responsibility by developing self-discipline and finishing what we start, always. I would not be a doctor had I never applied these principles to my own life. Sometimes, we stay away from getting involved or the "limelight" because we simply feel unqualified for the task at hand.

But here is the reality: those who make a difference in life or change the world do so not because they are necessarily the MOST qualified but simply because they DARED to DO something about their convictions! Remember in the scriptures, God never called someone because he or she was qualified for a job; rather He qualified them along the way. So keep this in mind as you read about how it is that such inequality came to be and how you can begin to be the force that alters the path.

We know that sex and gender play a role because medical experience has taught us many things, like autoimmune diseases are more common in women up to three times that of men, and that autism (another neurologic disease) seems to be much higher in men than women.[1] Yet, many clinicians and scientists continue to function in their practices of medicine, ignoring this basic knowledge—that sex and gender sometimes are directly intertwined with a presentation of a particular disease. Trying to diagnose and treat diseases ignoring these principles is like expecting a Boeing 747 to assemble itself by throwing all the right pieces onto a field.

In neurology, like in other medical fields, there are diseases more common in women than in men, like migraines, for instance.[2] Yet clinical trials have been male centric for years in all areas of medicine. According to the Journal of Women's Health (2006), women made up less than one-fourth of all patients enrolled in forty-six completed clinical trials in 2004. Some of the reasons cited for women being excluded date back to the 1950s. At the top of the list were birth defects to fetuses born to women who were or later became pregnant after participating in such trials like the thalidomide and DES drug studies.[3]

The drug thalidomide caused pregnant women to give birth to babies with serious birth defects (i.e., missing limbs). This trial was then followed by another drug trial with diethylstilbestrol, or DES, a synthetic nonsteroidal estrogen synthesized in 1938 designed to prevent miscarriages.[4] This, too, caused an increased risk of development of a rare vaginal cancer later in life for babies born to moms who partook of this drug. When these findings became known, both clinicians and drug companies became extremely cautious, with understandable concern. There was this inherent fear about possible unknown harm to fetuses of women that might become pregnant.

Subsequently, in 1977, partly in response to these tragedies, the FDA banned women who could become pregnant from participating in early-stage clinical trials. Unfortunately, in practice, the women who were banned became much more exclusive than previously anticipated or designed. Early-phase clinical trials broadened to ban not just women who were likely to conceive but rather the majority of women, including those who were homosexual, on contraceptives, or not sexually active. This ban lasted until 1993, when there were growing concerns about women's health issues being unaddressed.

Although the ban was eventually lifted, we still have a long way to go. In a study published in 2008 in the Journal of the American College of Cardiology, only 10 to 47% of each subject pool in nineteen heart-related trials consisted of women.[5] This is a hard blow considering the stark reality that more women die of heart disease than men each year! As an aside, despite this fact, most heart disease treatments are geared toward treating large-vessel disease common in men, while women have small-vessel disease, which is what is also commonly seen in stroke patients of different genders respectively. This is important to keep in mind because, if women have smaller vessel disease, in which high blood pressure is a big driving force, then medications, i.e., dopaminergic medications, that alter or influence this system could affect our risk factors for heart and brain disease and overall long-term health. (Note: there are no official studies to date on this subject looking at effects of dopamine medications as a risk factor for stroke and other cardiovascular diseases.) Still it is clear that women need to be properly represented in scientific studies to affect long-term positive change.

Congress passed the Revitalization Act that same year, 1993, mandating all NIH- (National Institute of Health) funded phase 3 trials to include women, unless exclusions were deemed appropriate. However, the problem of unbalanced research studies remains in most non-federally funded trials and has yet to be addressed by the FDA. Furthermore, many of the women who were allowed in trials were required to prove they would not get pregnant either via sterility or contraception prior to being admitted to particular studies. This practice was the norm in determining a woman's ability to participate in a trial in nearly 42% of 410 study protocols reviewed from 1994 to 1997, according to a published data in 2000 in Obstetrics & Gynecology.[6]

So, what then about pregnant women? And the YOPD patients who are of childbearing age? Will they not be represented in studies? This is the biggest challenge we are currently facing in order to be able to obtain the research data and studies that will help determine how many actual young women have PD and are having babies. Furthermore, we need to ascertain the medication risk for the mom and the fetus. Safety of DBS in pregnant women or those of childbearing age also remains unknown in the context of PD.

The fact is that Parkinson's women get pregnant (especially as many of us are starting to have families later in life or second families even) and pregnant women get Parkinson's. Previously some studies indicate there may be an increased risk to develop PD during pregnancy. But how are we to establish sound data and safe recommendations for our fellow women if we are not allowed to participate?

For instance, although one out of eight pregnant women takes an antidepressant[7], I speculate this might be higher within the pregnant Parkinson's population, since depression can be one of the presenting early symptoms of the disease—one-third of people with PD get depressed before PD is even diagnosed. These women are currently excluded from clinical trials in this field under the premise of "protecting fetuses from potential harm." One way of circumventing problems in regard to antidepressant medication effects on fetuses, and in particular in those mothers with Parkinson's, is to look at birth outcomes of women who are already on medication and become pregnant. Another alternative is to set up registries to evaluate a particular population, say, pregnant Parkinson's women.

Some drug companies already have registries for particular diseases like epilepsy or for certain drugs which treat specific diseases. Unfortunately, there are gaps both in communication, leaving many unaware of the existence of these registries—which means the information is never disseminated down to the patients who would be the ones to report to the registries besides the physicians—and in funding with smaller drug companies unable to afford to subsidize or maintain registries for their products.

Francoise Baylis, a professor of bioethics and philosophy at Dalhousie University in Canada, stated that one more disincentive for pharmaceutical companies to exclude pregnant women is a financial one. After all, "pregnant women are not considered to be a huge market (in the grand scheme of things), yet they carry a very large potential liability risk."[8] But we have to keep in mind that women are getting sicker, taking more medicines than ever, and starting families much later in life . . . when they are beginning to have a higher risk or higher risks for serious medical illnesses like neurodegenerative diseases such as PD.

Few new drugs are approved at present compared to previous years— all the new medicines released in the last several months are basically remakes, in my opinion, or remodeling of already existing ones. The reason for this paucity of novel (i.e. new) drugs has to do with a large number of them failing in clinical trials in early phases, and also because many trials never get filled. I believe if we were to open all phases of clinical trials to those who in years past have been excluded, such as minorities and females, perhaps we could avoid some of the last decade's disappointments. This belief is backed by the Society for Women's Health Research, founded in 1990 to champion the women's issues in healthcare reform. They discovered that although sanctions have been repealed on paper by the government and NIH, women continue to be excluded out of most trials, particularly in early phase clinical studies.[9] However, in order for women's issues to be fully addressed, scientists need to do more than just meet sex quotas in trials and studies. Researchers must begin to frame questions from a woman's perspective, taking into account her needs and background. As Ruth Faden, executive director of John Hopkins Berman Institute of Bioethics, has said: scientists need to realize that we "[PD] women are NOT [just] mirror images of PD men minus the penises,"[10] because not only do we have completely different chemical compositions than men, but even when we do have the same identical composition, as in identical twins, there still is no guarantee that both will develop disease. In fact, studies have shown that Parkinson's patients who have an identical or a fraternal twin have the same risk of getting PD as the general population.[11]

Tragically, although the world has moved forward in its view of the role of women in society, it seems that within the confines of medicine and science, we are still operating in an archaic world, even though according to recent data of medical school applicants, the distribution of male students to female is nearly half.[(12)]

The way you and I can influence science is by getting involved. There are many ways in which your contribution to the science could be vital, from participating in clinical trials to sitting on committees and boards that review study protocols which will take women's perspective and issues into account. Today's research and tomorrows treatments ARE in the palm of your hand! You may want to start by joining me and many others like me in becoming a research advocate for Parkinson's. You may want to start this process by becoming part of the Parkinson's Disease Foundation's (PDF's) Parkinson's Advocate in Research (PAIR) program, which teaches individuals the necessary skills to "pair up" with scientists and health professionals in the community to bring about change. You can also sign up to become an "e-advocate" for the Parkinson's Action Network (PAN), which is the organization that deals with influencing and transforming ideas in healthcare into laws that impact all of our lives, especially in the area of neurology research and Parkinson's disease awareness and care.

"Be the change you want to see in the world" is one of the driving forces behind my pursuit for a better living experience, which includes new treatments for all those who deal with Parkinson's on a daily basis. We all have been given different talents for a unique purpose. I encourage everyone to use their special gifts to reach out to others in whatever capacity they can, whether as active research participants, or by driving others who cannot get to research centers or in an opportunity to participate themselves. You and only you are the expert of your disease; therefore, you can educate others, to push for changes in healthcare, or make way for new technologies like devices to help with gait or eating. A personal story can be more empowering and relatable than any medical lecture. Become an active advocate if just within your own community. Be creative. Be the change.

You are more than equipped for new roles and challenges. Here are several ways in which you might be able to participate:

- Enroll in a research study.
- Invite scientists in your area to come and meet with Parkinson's patients in the community (round-table discussion).
- Give talks on the importance of research participation and female involvement especially.
- Speak with your physicians about opportunities to work with them in research planning (see if they would welcome a female patient perspective).
- Write letters to your congressmen and senators about issues important to the PD community, particularly those affecting women and minorities.
- Become an active member of the Parkinson's Action Network (PAN) and PAIR, previously mentioned. PAN is the unified voice of the Parkinson's community advocating for better treatments, quality of life, and a cure. This will keep you up-to-date on latest developments as well as important issues involving healthcare impacting our PD community.
- Don't forget to thank your neurologists/movement disorder specialists for their sticking-to-it-iveness in this current national healthcare crisis brought on by the passing of the Affordable Care Act, which has led to much interference with doctors' old ways of practicing medicine, driving many physicians away from their fields because they are no longer able to make ends meet due to government cutbacks on reimbursements. Without their dedication and valiant work, we Parkinson's patients would be lost. Write them a thank you card reminding them why they matter and how they are making a difference in your life.

For me, research, whether clinical or basic science, has been part of my repertoire since I was in college, working in a lab involving transgenic mice and setting my own research protocols to studying schizophrenic patients as part of my undergraduate studies. Later, as a neurology resident, I was part of several research studies. While I was in private practice, it was exciting to see novel drugs come out, particularly those in which I had an active part, either as a researcher or participant. The new medications provided me with an increased armamentarium to combat the disease, and it gave me the confidence that what I was prescribing for my patients was not only safe, but efficacious as well. Both as part of my training and in my solo practice, I conducted several research studies reinforcing my passion for my chosen field, even though there was a time when my friends thought I was crazy for wanting to go into a field once known for its lack of treatments. This was jokingly referred to as a "Diagnose and Adios" type of specialty, due to the fact that at the time of my entering the neurology field, the last medication had been introduced at least thirty years earlier.

Despite the naysayers, I followed my heart, and to this day, I still believe in the promise of a better tomorrow for those who suffer many neurological illnesses like Parkinson's. The hope is to one day find a cure for Parkinson's. With your help and participation and with our growing scientific knowledge, which can be molded and inspired by you, we CAN find a CURE! Until that time, please join me in my quest and stand proud at being called dreamers . . .

After all, it is the dreamers who possess the exorbitant imagination that underlines the power behind the changes in our world.

2

History & Symptoms of Parkinson's Disease

SHAKING PALSY (Paralysis Agitans)
"Involuntary tremulous motion, with lessened muscular power,
in parts not in action and even when supported; with a propen-
sity to bend the trunk forwards, and to pass from a walking to
a running pace; the senses and intellects being uninjured." [1, 2]
~ James Parkinson

Although Parkinson's disease bears its name after a British surgeon by the name of James Parkinson, who published the "Essay on the Shaking Palsy" in 1817, many others before him had described similar symptoms. The first record of note was made sometime in the second century A.D. by a great Greek physician known as Galen.[3] He has been credited with distinguishing tremors at rest from other types of tremors. Dr. John Hunter, who was a renowned surgeon, lecturer, and meticulous record-keeper, compiled a complete description of this illness, which some speculate was the driving force for Dr. Parkinson to begin his observation and notations of several people walking at the park who possessed what we now know to be the characteristic clinical findings of the disease.[4, 5, 6] However, long before the famous French neurologist by the name of Jean-Martin Charcot insisted the disease bear the name of Parkinson's disease in honor of Dr. Parkinson, which may very well be the "only time in history the French ever credited the Brits for anything," as a colleague once quipped. Being a Francophile myself, I believe he is absolutely correct! However, prior to this, there were many descriptions of a similar disease in ancient Egypt and ancient India dating back as early as the tenth century BC.[7] Although the term "Parkinson's disease" was coined by Charcot, most of the understanding regarding the pathology and chemical involvement occurred at least eighty years after the "Essay on the Shaking Palsy" was first published. And even though the isolation of dopamine as the primary neurotransmitter involved in the disease did not occur until the 1950s, an ancient Indian civilization over two thousand years old was ahead of its time. This civilization, in their Ayurveda medical treatise, which clearly described an illness involving tremors, drooling lack of movement, and other symptoms we now associate with PD, treated people suffering from these symptoms with remedies from the Mucuna family, which is rich in levodopa (L-dopa).[8, 9]

Although we presume that the compound consumed back in ancient times was that specifically of Mucuna pruriens, known as Atmagupta in Sanskrit,[10] we don't know exactly how much or how it was given as remedy for this ailment, even though we could probably make some educated guesses. In Central America, particularly in Brazil, these "velvet beans" have been roasted for decades to make a coffee substitute we know as Nescafe. Single portions of about an ounce of the seeds have been shown to be as effective as single doses of modern Parkinson's medicines. However, long-term efficacy and tolerability have not been established as of yet.[11] A few studies have attempted to replicate the validity and efficacy of this natural product as a possible viable treatment for modern-day Parkinson's disease. What we know so far is that, in large amounts (i.e., 30 g dose), it has been shown to be as effective as pure Sinemet (levodopa/carbidopa) in the treatment of PD. However, no known long-term efficacy and tolerability data is available.[12] This would seem like an ideal treatment, since it not only is rich in dopamine but also contains serotonin, another chemical often responsible for some of the non-motor symptoms of PD. In several phase 3 trials, this cowage (Mucuna pruriens), a bean-like plant, which grows wild in the tropics including India and southern Florida, was found to be just as potent as levodopa and did not increase dyskinesia. Researchers found that 30 g of this bean had a much more rapid onset of action and lasted longer without increasing dyskinesia.[13] One small study even showed faster improvement in motor fluctuations with Mucuna 30 mg than Sinemet 50/200.[14]

At present time, there are no recommended doses since further studies are needed. Even though the active compound found in these seeds is exactly the same as the standard medicine, and therefore, side effects would be the same as with L-dopa, we have to remember that these seeds also contain other compounds like serotonin, etc. These other naturally occurring chemicals in the plant could be the source for their effectiveness, while at the same time; these could pose potential added side effects and interaction with other medications. In addition, these seeds are not currently regulated by the FDA. Thus, any single brand may be lacking in the purity or strength claimed on the label, which could lead to toxicity or ineffectiveness.

If you were to use Mucuna, first discuss with your healthcare provider. Never make any changes without your provider's consent. If your doctor agrees to allow this as a trial, look for supplements labeled "USP verified" to ensure potency, bioavailability, and purity of the cowage seed. Finally, remember that these are foreign substances, like any other prescribed medication, even if natural, with potentially harmful side effects. Therefore, this treatment is not recommended without the direction and guidance of your physician. We know from ancient scripts and small trials that this naturally occurring bean plant indeed has healing powers, but we don't know to what extent the effects were due to its natural dopamine component alone or in combination with the natural serotonin it also holds within. In theory, this may be the ideal medication; this may be the ideal treatment targeting both motor and non-motor symptoms simultaneously. Only time will tell.

I often wonder if the ancient civilizations were any closer to a cure with their holistic approaches. For sure, we have been in the business of replacing dopamine in sufferers for more than half a century, and although we have made great strides in the treatment of PD, I can't help but wonder what it is about dopamine that keeps us talking about it ad nauseum. I have been hearing the same arguments for over twenty-five years, while I was still a college student and long before I became a Parkinson's specialist, and longer yet before I had to learn to live with the disease myself. Is it better to be given continuously or in bursts? Is it toxic or neuroprotective (i.e., good for the longevity of the brain)? Maybe it's time we realized that dopamine may be the oldest but not the ONLY child of our brains, so we should start paying attention to its siblings, such as serotonin, and more importantly, the interaction between them, which may hold the key to a cure.

Four main motor symptoms of Parkinson's:[15]

Rest tremors
Gait instability
Muscle stiffness
Slowness (of movements)

Other non-motor symptoms:

Loss of smell
Anxiety/depression
Constipation
Sleep disorders/restless leg/ REM behavior
Memory loss/ cognitive problems
Pain
Fatigue
Bladder problems
Visual problems

Risk factors:

Advancing age
Male gender
Decreased estrogen /early hysterectomy with ovary removal
Environmental toxins
Agricultural workers, well water consumption
Repeat (frequent) head trauma or severe head injury

Other lesser known risk factors:
Hispanic ethnicity
Family or personal history of essential tremors
Family history of Parkinson's
History of restless leg or REM behavior (acting out dreams when body is supposed to be paralyzed)
History of anxiety/mood disorders
History of chronic constipation
Migraine with aura (in middle age women)

The typical Parkinson's patient is over the age of fifty-five and comprises 90-95% of the Parkinson's population. This is idiopathic Parkinson's disease. Young onset Parkinson's disease (YOPD) presents itself prior to age forty and makes up about 5-10% of the Parkinson's population. YOPD has not been well understood, until recently, thanks to social media and other forms of mass communication. Now we are getting a closer look into a disease that continues to baffle even the experts.

In the United States, there are nearly 1.5 million people living with this condition, and countless others who dedicate their lives to caring for PD patients, which is estimated to be around seven million people worldwide. Look around you. You may be surprised to find many of these individuals living in your community. The financial burden of Parkinson's, not to mention the social and emotional devastation which is ever increasing as the disease progresses, leaves many of these patients and their families isolated and destitute.

The more we are willing to open our heart and minds to learn, the better equipped we can be at helping our friends and neighbors who struggle with this chronic, deteriorating brain disease, characterized by loss of a "black substance," called the substancia nigra deep in the area of the brain known as the basal ganglia. Here in this area is where the chemical dopamine, which was first identified by Arvid Carlsson in the 1950s[16], is found. Loss of this important neurotransmitter (a messenger that sends signals to various other brain cells) is what leads to the symptoms of Parkinson's mentioned above. This chemical, which gives the black color to the substancia nigra, is responsible for fine motor movements, coordination, muscle control, as well being as a key player in the reward- and pleasure-seeking center of the brain. For years after the development of Sinemet in the late 1960s, scientists and neurologists improved the lives of many suffering from this illness by prescribing this medication, which still remains the gold standard of treatment. However, we know that dopamine is not the only chemical involved in Parkinson's disease. If it was as simple as just replacing dopamine, we would have likely found a cure by now. Dopamine was an extraordinary accomplishment that has taught us much about the disease and its chemical properties. This chemical has properties which cause brain cells to thrive, and it induces survival, development, and function of neurons. Furthermore, when dopamine is administered to Parkinson's patients, it has been shown to reduce the rate of death, thus putting to rest a long-held myth that dopamine/L-dopa was toxic to neurons and patients.[17, 18]

So, what is the take-home from all this?

The sooner a patient can begin treatment, the better. I still encounter people who are simply panicked about taking medications because of the fear of side effects and potential for dyskinesia, certainly legitimate concerns. Still, when patients are armed with knowledge about Parkinson's and their options, they can make better choices for themselves.

Postponing dopamine treatment only hurts the patient in the long run. By starting medications earlier, patients have been shown to have a better outcome and extended quality of life compared to those who delay treatment.[19]

Notwithstanding the advances in treatments in recent years, there appears to be a rise in both incidence (the number of new cases in a single year in a given area) and prevalence (how widespread a disease, in this case Parkinson's, is in the population in a given geographical area) of typical idiopathic PD, particularly as the population ages. Of note, I have observed the same trend in YOPD, but to date epidemiological studies have not been carried out to document these trends in the general population. According to Dorsey et al., the PD population over fifty years of age is expected to double by year 2030 in the US to 600,000.[20] However, we are not alone. As other countries become industrialized and improve their healthcare systems, they too are expected to see an increase in the duration and length of illness.[21] Awareness of the disease and its associated societal burden are crucial so that we may begin to shape appropriate treatment strategies that are not only gender specific but socially appropriate within the context of each individual race or ethnic group, particularly when Parkinson's seems to be so individualized. However, this is only on the surface. In reality, if you start looking closer at various cross-sections of the Parkinson's population, general patterns begin to emerge, especially within genders. We must begin to preplan for the benefit of patients and their loved ones, and to demand from our governments, health professionals, and research institutes like the National Institute of Health (NIH), not just excellence of care but appropriate policies to care for these increased number of patients and their affected families in which the primary goal is improvement in quality of daily living.

If you believe to have any of the symptoms of Parkinson's, please seek the advice of a healthcare professional immediately. Although there are no blood tests to confirm the diagnosis of Parkinson's, work still continues in an attempt to find a biomarker to easily identify those at risk of disease early on. However, I believe, as do many others in my field, that under the care of a specialist such as a neurologist or a movement disorder specialist, the diagnosis itself can be accurate up to 95% of the time under the right circumstances, meaning the patients present with a typical or common clinical pattern physicians recognize as Parkinson's. Of note, specialists have a broader clinical spectrum of knowledge because they see all the various stages and presentations of an illness and are more apt to recognize something as being typical for the disease when someone else who does have similar experience might not. Additionally, in the hands of a specialist, a PD patient's quality of life can be vastly improved, despite the fact there is no cure. An experienced specialist can detect subtle changes and institute appropriate measures early on, such as involving other ancillary services and other specialists to ensure the best outcome possible via a team approach.

3

Parkinson's Disease Presentation Varies Depending on Age of Onset and Gender

"Man cannot live on chocolate alone, but women sure can."
~ Author Unknown

With PD on the rise, gender differences in PD are extremely important to review, understand, and consider, given the huge implications for future generations of women treatment plans. The success or failure of their outcomes will have a great impact not only on their descendants if they are of childbearing age but also on social planning.

In treating women with PD, we should take into account women's needs when considering their plan of care.

- Are they of childbearing age?
- Are they breastfeeding?
- Are they a caregiver to others?
- Will they have help from others if they get pregnant and experience a worsening of their symptoms during the pregnancy?

Even if gender and hormonal differences turn out not to be a factor, I think looking at sex differences merits at least some consideration, especially in light of the fact that we know hormones/gender play a role in women's illnesses, making us more likely to get migraines, have autoimmune diseases, have more side effects from medications than men, and twice as likely to be depressed than men.[1, 2, 3]

Hence, Parkinson's disease should not be looked at in a two-dimensional form but in three dimensions, in which being a woman plays a bigger role in not just any illness but particularly those of chronic progressive nature such as PD. Women with Parkinson's, especially when young, can and do often present with different (non-traditional symptoms) than their male counterparts. We know for a fact that women prior to menopause have completely different symptoms when having a heart attack, with symptoms that mimic almost anything under the sun, and since young women are not readily considered to be at risk for coronary heart disease, they are often misdiagnosed and untreated. Once women become menopausal, the risk of having a heart attack line up to those of their male counterparts. So, I ask myself if we are misdiagnosing or missing young onset Parkinson's in women for the same reason. We need to begin looking beyond what is in front of us and consider the whole. I encourage all health professionals to look at the patient's gender as well as their hormonal status, not just for clues to diagnosis, but more importantly, once a diagnosis is confirmed, to guide appropriate treatment plans. After all, have we ever known men and women to behave the same or respond the same to stress, whether internal or external?

Ever since my first encounter with that young Hispanic female during my residency (see Preface), I have been intrigued by these thoughts:

- Why would women be affected at a young age?
- What triggered the disease at an early age versus an older age?
- Is young onset Parkinson's different than the more common idiopathic Parkinson's?
- Are there gender differences in PD such as I have observed in other neurological and medical diseases?
- Do hormones play a role?

It has been more than twenty years since my first encounter with the young Hispanic woman. Since then, I was in practice for a good number of years and treated a lot of women with PD, which included a fair number of young women with Parkinson's. One thing is for certain, at least in my experience; the women with young onset PD never behaved like the older typical PD patients. Through the years, I have always kept a mental note of these differences in the back of my mind and have been extremely puzzled by this observation, to the point that I thought it was time to put into writing.

As the saying goes, *"There are no rainbows without storms!"* It turns out that any perceived rainstorms would pale in comparison to the huge thunderstorm that was about to take over my life.

Up to that point, I had devoted my life to working with Parkinson's patients and others with movement disorders.

Gradually, I began noticing that I was beginning to exhibit some of the *same* symptoms as the patients I was examining! I, too, had Parkinson's disease!

As dumbfounded and somewhat apprehensive about my future as I was, having knowledge of all the intricacies of the disease firsthand was helpful. As a Parkinson's specialist, I also realized I was not dealing with a typical scenario. Yes, I had the stiffness, slowness, and gait problems, but only very little if any rest tremors. Even now, eight years into the disease, rest tremors are not very prominent for me and, in fact, are more pronounced in my left foot than in my hand. Other peculiar characteristics that I presented with at onset of my illness, aside from depression and anxiety, was severe pain and visual disturbances. But my formal training dictated I should have all four main features in some shape or form. Yet, I was missing a big component of the disease, the rest tremors, plus I had other symptoms not typical of Parkinson's disease. Nevertheless, my personal experience in treating young women with PD over the years had taught me to expect a different presentation in YOPD. So in my heart of hearts, I knew I had PD by some ironic twist of fate, although my formal training insisted this could not be so—not enough evidence. Or at least I was secretly praying that my instincts were way off base this time!

After much deliberation between my husband, who firmly believed I was simply overworked and identifying too much with my patients, and a number of specialists, who kept shrugging their shoulders, making me even more anxious, I finally had to call upon a dear friend, whom I trusted completely. I approached my visit with her in complete honesty. Since she had worked with me as a resident and knew me well as a person, physician, and friend, I felt she could be the one person to set me straight. After many dead ends, I asked the question in my husband's mind: was I just too stressed and identifying with the patients I loved? My friend, colleague and movement disorder specialist informed me that *yes*, much to my chagrin, my problem was **indeed in my brain** rather than in my head! The news came both as a vindication that I was not crazy, that I did know my neurology and still had a strong medical intuition, but with a heavy heart knowing the implications of the diagnosis. Although the question of visual disturbances was still unresolved in both our minds, we opted to start treatment with levodopa. To my and my doctor's astonishment, the visual problems had an obvious and dramatic response to levodopa, as did the pain.

Looking back at my own YOPD patients, in general they had little in the way of rest tremors, presented with dystonia (involuntary sustained contractions of the muscles), and frequently had more depression and anxiety, which at times seemed out of proportion to their disease. Few of them had visual disturbances as I did, which neither I nor my fellow colleagues were able to correlate at the time to PD. Like other Parkinson's specialists at the time, I spent most of my time focusing on the motor aspects of the disease and documenting such changes via the UPDRS (Unified Parkinson's Disease Rating Scale), which measures motor fluctuations. Unfortunately, I feel that because of lack of understanding of non-motor symptoms and YOPD, some of my female patients' complaints were not attributed to PD. It is a travesty to think of those whose main complaints were things like anxiety and depression in the face of no tremors and slight motor problems, to an untrained eye, would have been perceived as normal. We now understand that non-motor symptoms like depression, anxiety, constipation, sleep disorders, bladder problems, and loss of smell can precede motor symptoms up to twenty years[4, 5], and this includes less commonly known and understood symptoms like pain, fatigue, and visual disturbances.[6, 7, 8] Not until the last five to ten years were these non-motor symptoms considered to be a part of the PD clinical picture; since then, our understanding of non-motor symptoms in PD has skyrocketed. Recent studies have shown that 40% of PD patients at onset have fatigue, independent of depression, daytime sleepiness, or motor difficulties, while a whopping 40-80% experience pain, with pain being the second most common problem encountered by patients after mobility issues.[9] The combination of pain and fatigue can be devastating to anyone's life and much more if that person is suffering from a chronic illness already. So very few people to date, and even fewer yet in the medical profession, have grasped the concept of pain being a huge factor in PD. Pain, if not recognized or undertreated, will not only limit a person's ability to carry on activities of daily living but also will cause severe emotional damage, leading to depression, apathy and hopelessness.

Subsequently, I have spent much of my time since my diagnosis trying to educate myself anew regarding the latest theories, research, and so on. Interestingly enough, slowly over the same amount of time, scientists and neurologists and MDS (motor disorder specialists) have moved from thinking of PD as a purely central nervous system disorder into thinking of it as more of a systemic disease, involving not only the dopamine system but also many other systems, like the serotonin system, etc. We now know that it is the deficits in these other systems that account for these less commonly known symptoms like pain, fatigue, sleep disorders, and depression. The presence of non-motor symptoms is gradually becoming more acceptable although still poorly understood. Still, little is known or understood as to why PD patients present with such varying symptoms. Thus, my question remains: is there a difference in presentation among men and women with PD due to their gender or age of onset?

When I began pulling the ideas for this book together, there was not a lot of data regarding gender differences in Parkinson's disease, and much research still needs to be done. However, slowly, like the grains of sand through an hourglass, we are at the brink of great new discoveries and unveiling new fundamental principles, which will forever once more shape the lives of those with PD, as it was in 1987 when Alim Benabid first discovered the potentials of high-frequency stimulation to the thalamus.[10] Not entirely a novel idea. Dr. Charcot in the nineteenth century had devised a vibratory chair for his PD patients after observing that they slept better and their symptoms improved transiently after a train, boat, or carriage ride. His junior protégé, Gilles de la Tourette, went a step further and devised a vibrating helmet, resembling a Viking's helmet, which provided external stimulation to the brain, based on the premise that the brain would respond better to direct stimulation. However, his theories were not pursued until the twenty-first century.[11]

The thalamus is a deep-brain structure named for its appearance derived from the Greek word "inner chamber," or "sleeping room" in Latin, because it has two lobes which are intricately connected.[12] These lobes are involved in control of movement as well as sensory function, which includes pain. When Benabid stimulated this area, it caused tremors to subside, leading to medical applications of deep brain stimulation (DBS).[13] Although this wonderful technology has been available for years, it seems as if few have truly benefited from the treatment. First of all, it has taken almost twenty years for the PD community to become aware of its existence, and in my experience, is offered less to women with PD. In fact, women with PD are 30% less likely than men to obtain DBS, and if you are a woman in a minority group, your chances are even less: African Americans and Asians received 80% and 45%, respectively, less DBS treatments compared to white beneficiaries.[14]

The reason?

There are a number of recent studies that show women act and present differently than men when it comes to Parkinson's disease. Perhaps it is these differences in presentation that are keeping us from obtaining time-proven effective treatment.

Why do women act differently in the face of PD? There has been a long debate that states maybe estrogen is to blame. Some say it is because estrogen plays a "brain cell protector" role in PD as it does in other neurological diseases, such as strokes and Alzheimer's[15], so as long as we women have our hormones, we have a decreased chance of getting PD. For example, getting an early hysterectomy with removal of ovaries has been shown to increase the risk of Parkinson's in women[16] I will venture to say that if hormones, especially estrogen, are not neuroprotective in nature—in other words, not in the best interest of keeping brain cells functioning normally—at the very least, they are involved in the safekeeping of the brain and body against degeneration.

I also suggest that hormones are a big factor for why we see a wide variation in PD presentation, including age of onset, between men and women, but more importantly why women with PD seem to be more prone to develop "negative" outcomes (such as job loss due to symptoms and a general discontent with quality of life) as well as an increase in non-motor symptoms, such as depression.[17, 18] Clearly, when dealing with stressors, men are from Venus and women are from Mars, as they say. Many women, including myself at times, when the injury is grave, tend to cry out in rage, frustration, hurt, and sadness until the tears wash away all the pain. For me, only when I have given in to my sorrow for a time am I able to focus and begin again. For women, by not dealing with what frightens us, such as an incurable disease like PD, and letting out our frustrations and tears, we only build a scab around our wounds, which we constantly protect, and therefore, we cannot move forward. While men usually are more stoic with their emotions, bottling it all up and ignoring them, tending to let worries either pile on or roll on by. Perhaps this is one of the reasons why men with PD have many more behavioral issues compared to women with PD. Men with PD, unlike women with PD, tend to have more aggression, exhibiting abusive behavior, both verbal and physical, and are at greater risk of wandering. Therefore, they are more likely to be placed on antipsychotics, whereas the women are more likely to receive antidepressants. For the males, perhaps this behavior is their way of acting out frustrations and releasing their pent-up anger.[19]

Yet, the role of estrogen in Parkinson's disease remains controversial to say the least, muddled by various confounding factors like intake of birth control pills and number of years a woman has taken contraceptives. The correlation between years of contraceptive intake and risk of Parkinson's is not a linear; however, much work remains to be done in this area to look for other factors predisposing women to PD besides undergoing an early hysterectomy with oophorectomy, that is to say removal of the uterus along with ovaries, where the ovaries seem to be the key. If this surgical procedure takes place before menopause, there appears to be an increased risk of developing Parkinsonism, by as much as 68% in those women. [20] As I have stated previously, we cannot entirely dismiss the potential beneficial role of estrogen in PD as it is seen in other neurological and medical diseases, like strokes and heart disease. A ten-year study in which 119,166 postmenopausal women ages fifty to seventy-one were surveyed regarding their hormone replacement therapy (HRT) revealed that taking contraceptives for over ten years versus not taking contraceptives was associated with a lower PD risk. Researchers also found that use of menopausal HRT in women for less than five years revealed a higher risk of PD compared to those who did not use hormone supplements. [21] Although at first these findings may seem contradictory, they reinforce the fact of a definitive role for estrogen and oxytocin in risk of PD, and they speak of the importance of timing as to when hormones should be replaced or withdrawn, such as with the removal of the ovaries. This timing is imperative for us to master as far as when hormone replacement might be more detrimental or beneficial to our brain's function. [22]

This idea is based on the theory of a positive effect of HRT around the time of menopause also known as the "timing hypothesis." [23] This concept was initially described in the context of lack of heart disease from HRT when instituted close to menopause in the Women's Health Initiative Study. [24] The idea arose from the "critical window" hypothesis, which says that estrogen therapy, when initiated early in menopause, can be beneficial for the brain; on the other hand, if added later in menopause, it can be harmful or ineffective. [25, 26]

So, yes! At least from what we know so far, hormones do play a vital role in women's PD issues. For instance, we know from limited studies that when women with PD become pregnant, they can experience an exacerbation of their symptoms. Fortunately, these symptoms were reported to be self-limited, resolving after delivery.[27, 28]

Furthermore, we women are not just subject to the hormonal influences which set us apart from our male counterparts, but we also are more likely to develop dyskinesia (Greek for difficulty in movement or impairment in the ability to control movements, resulting in fragmented or jerky movements), particularly if we develop Parkinsonism at any age. [29, 30] But independent of age, women are more likely to experience more dyskinesias on average than men with PD as a group.[31]

Even though all of us, men and women, release the same type of hormones (we will discuss more on these in a later chapter) during stress, both genders respond to stress in different ways. The reason for these differences between the sexes has to do with the degree of concentration of one particular hormone, known as oxytocin.[32] These differences are especially significant, since the buildup of oxytocin usually leads to a reduction in the impact of dopamine and serotonin in our brains.[33] Thus, when it comes to stress and Parkinson's, it appears that we women are predisposed to a "double whammy effect," in which stress releases oxytocin, which in turn lowers our already low or depleted dopamine systems, which in turn makes us more vulnerable to experiencing apathy, depression, and other negative symptoms compared to our male Parkinson's friends.

To recap, we have so far discussed how the differences in levels of estrogen and oxytocin between men and women could possibly account for variations in the presentation of PD symptoms between the sexes, as well as throughout the illness. Women with YOPD tend to have painful cramps and rigidity more commonly upon presentation, as was the case with my initial presentation, making me, in fact, rather typical for my age group and gender. The same holds true for most of the young women whom I have personally diagnosed in my years in practice and in those whom I have observed through my role as a research advocate for the Parkinson's Disease Foundation.

Yet, the few studies available on women appeared to contradict my own experience. In these studies, women were found to have more tremors.[34] I suspect there is collection bias in these studies because women of all ages are lumped together. Older PD women may present with tremor as do their male counterparts, but young PD women who don't normally present with tremors are NOT given a diagnosis until the tremor is seen—therefore making it seem like tremor is the presenting symptom for all women. I believe more studies are necessary to further evaluate. However, if we were indeed to believe that women with Parkinson's do have MORE tremors than men and having tremor-dominant Parkinson's disease holds a better prognosis typically since it usually progresses slower, then why are PD women more disabled than men with this disease?

We must try to find a way to correct these discrepancies in disabilities, which lean more heavily toward those of us of the feminine persuasion. One way is to establish social work programs, along with greater number of women support groups and access to counseling geared toward empowering women, teaching them to be self-advocates, and learning tools necessary to help navigate the challenges we face on a daily basis as women trying to balance families, careers, and Parkinson's. Only as we become masters of our own destinies can we successfully find a way to break the stress cycle caused by the physical and emotional state induced by our illness.

I am glad that there are now groups forming for the sole purpose of lifting up the Parkinson's woman's spirit, to offer aid, to teach coping skills, and to reinforce a person's values for who they are on the inside. One such group is the Women's Parkinson's Support Group run by Darcy Blake out of Palo Alto, California (www.parkinsonswomen.com). The reason many of us women become disabled is because we tend to lose our support systems, leaving many of us destitute with nowhere and no one to turn to, increasing our inner oxytocin levels due to stress, depleting our brain's dopamine faster, all in a vicious, downward-spiraling cycle. We already have our cards stacked against us even before we get diagnosis. As I mentioned we are more prone to depression than men and this is worse during our menstrual cycle, pregnancies and during menopause.[35] Add PD into the mix, where the rate of depression is as high as 80%, and no wonder we PD women as a group are top consumers of antidepressants.[36, 37] Although incidents of depression in PD patients appear to be independent of age of diagnosis, it is much more significant and pronounced if a woman has young onset Parkinson's.[38]

So women with PD are more likely to develop depression, dyskinesia, and anxiety, and have hormonal influences due to stress patterns and menstrual-cycle changes caused by PD. Conversely, when a woman is menstruating, Parkinson's symptoms can become worse—the fatigue, tremors, stiffness, and so on. We are creatures bound by our hormones.[39] I suppose that, because of the hormonal changes, menstrual changes, and the sedentary life a depressed person might assume, women with PD tend to exhibit a higher risk for hip fractures, with an estimated 7.3% lower bone mineral density compared to those who don't have PD.[40]

The greatest risk of experiencing a hip fracture was documented in older Parkinson's women, especially those over the age of sixty-five—as high as 10.4%.[41] Perhaps the reason we see an increased risk as we age is due to a multifactorial, cumulative effect from (1) loss of estrogen that occurs as we age, which worsens after menopause, causing osteoporosis; (2) loss of vitamin D, which occurs with Parkinson's disease; (3) decreased mobility; and (4) decreased sun light exposure. Add to that other common medical problems of the elderly, like diabetes, thyroid disease, peripheral neuropathies, and poor vision and hearing, which combined results in loss of balance. Finally, consider B12 deficiency which is common in Parkinson's and could be disaster waiting to happen if not properly diagnosed and managed on time! Parkinson's patients must take the initiative to mitigate falls and hip fractures by drinking dairy products, replacing vitamin D and B12 levels if low, exercising routinely to strengthen bones and getting sunlight exposure several times a week —morning is preferred time for optimal results.[42]

This preventive plan of care is important due to the fact that people with PD who undergo hip surgery do not fare as well as non-PD patients during surgery and in recovery.[43, 44] This prevention-oriented initiative may include hormonal supplementation, if your doctor deems it necessary and there are no contraindications. Most important is measuring bone density in YOPD women at an earlier age than that recommended by FDA or Medicare, etc., which means your doctor will have to document reasons for needing the bone scan. I get a bone scan every two years. After all, women as a gender are four times more likely to develop osteoporosis independent of Parkinson's disease.[45] By closely watching bone density levels, we hope to prevent hip fractures and unnecessary hospitalizations and surgeries, which will only add to anxiety and stress.

As a neurologist who treated Parkinson's patients for years, I know that certain neurological diseases have dramatic presentation differences and treatment options based on gender. After many centuries, we are now beginning to get a sense that gender does matter in the face of Parkinson's disease too. By understanding the subtleties of gender differences and variations in presentation according to age of onset within the Parkinson's spectrum, doctors and patients could then be able to optimize their therapeutic care and significantly improve their quality of life.

My desire is that these cues will jumpstart a new set of guidelines for Parkinson's treatments that measures the risks and needs according to each patient's gender, age, and hormonal status, including menstrual cycle, to make better-informed decisions for our patients, ourselves, and our loves ones.

4

Misdiagnosing PD in Young Women

"I don't think inside the box, I don't think OUTSIDE the box,
I don't EVEN KNOW where the box is!"

~ Author Unknown

Parkinson's disease is typically found in people over the age of fifty with a less common form presenting in those less than forty years of age, which can extend into the early twenties, known as young onset Parkinson's disease (YOPD)[1]. There is yet a third type, an even rarer form than YOPD, known as Juvenile Parkinson's Disease, affecting teens and children, which for the sake of this book will not be discussed.

Diagnosing Parkinson's in a young person is not an easy feat, even for those of us who have a bit more experience delivering a diagnosis of PD. This is true not only because of the rarity of YOPD, but also because of the atypical, or not so straightforward, presentation compared to idiopathic Parkinson's disease. However, I firmly believe that the cases of YOPD, or at least Parkinsonism, are increasing in number, both here in the states and around the world. The reason for this apparent increase in incidence is not yet known nor do we have quantifiable data to prove this. Still, if the incidence is on the rise as I suspect, it is probably due to a number of factors colliding all at once.

We know that most of Parkinson's is idiopathic, meaning "cause unknown," and only about 10% of those with PD are familial or genetic in nature.[2] We also know that there are several environmental factors, like toxins, which influence a person who might already be "predisposed" to develop the disease.[3] It is my opinion that some of these known toxins, such as pesticides added to our produce and growth hormones implemented in the feeding of livestock and other animals like chickens, may be wreaking havoc on our hormones, thus increasing a woman's tendency to have PD especially at a younger age. Furthermore, I contend that epidemiological studies have not captured the full spectrum or the severity of the disease to date, leaving large unanswered gaps among the young, socioeconomically challenged and the various minority groups of our society. These factors could possibly contribute to a delay in seeking healthcare among those with PD, causing a trickledown effect of exclusion and under-diagnosis in these subgroups.[4]

Perhaps because of the reasons above or some other factor we are yet to discover, women with PD are still lagging behind, taking much longer from onset of first symptom to having that first visit with a movement disorder specialist compared to the men with PD—it is in fact 61% longer.[5] I believe the reason for these lagtimes has to do with established subconscious prejudices within the medical field. At times, during the practice of medicine, we as physicians may become fixed and rigid within the scope of our training, and we must be willing to recondition our brains to think outside the box, to allow for the changes in neuroscience that may go beyond our own preconceived notions and expectations. In the case of Parkinson's disease, pieces of the puzzle are still missing. Perhaps we need to start looking at PD in terms of gender and ethnicity to see the whole picture. Although at present time, epidemiology studies suggests that Parkinson's is more common in older white males; this may change once we consider different ethnicities and look at gender in more detail.

One of the limitations to diagnosis is lack of objective blood testing. So, unless patients present with all four common signs right off the bat *and* are of the right age group (and, at times, gender), we as physicians may not even have Parkinson's disease on our radar. Hopefully, by the end of this book, all of us, whether lay persons or health professionals, will at least begin to think of PD in new ways, including the differential diagnoses of a young person who presents without rest tremors, but with pain, fatigue, depression, visual disturbances, olfactory problems, bladder dysfunction, constipation, sleep disorders, rigidity (stiffness of muscles), bradykinesia (Greek term which means slow movements), dystonia (abnormal involuntary sustained contraction of a muscles, i.e., writer's cramp), muscle cramping, and gait abnormalities.[6]

What makes diagnosis so challenging is the uniqueness of each individual's presentation. The key is learning to recognize patterns; this comes only from years of practice and seeing many patients of all stages. This is why it is so important to seek care from a specialist who sees hundreds of patients encompassing the entire spectrum of PD.

Another challenge to getting the right diagnosis is education through raising awareness both in the community as well in the health professional circuit. Unfortunately, in medicine as in any other walks of life, people tend to dismiss, trivialize, or label as "hysteria" what they don't know or fully comprehend. In the history of medicine, there are many examples of cases of diseases that we now recognize, particularly in the field of neurology, but were once dismissed or considered to be psychiatric disorders. In past centuries, the term "female hysteria"—from the Greek cognate relating to the uterus and, therefore, a women's problem—was a common label for women who presented with undefined symptoms. [7, 8] In ancient times, people believed those who experienced epileptic attacks to be possessed.[9] By the mid to late nineteenth century, the term "female hysteria," or "wandering womb," as it was also called, became known as a sexual dysfunction, and the general term of "hysteria" in 1980 was officially changed by the American Psychiatry Association to "conversion disorder."[10] "Conversion disorder" became a medical diagnosis widely prescribed to women for common ailments,[11] including faintness, muscle cramps; generalized malaise, sexual desires, loss of appetite, nervousness, insomnia, and fluid retention. These women were frequently characterized as difficult or "troublesome."[12] Although the terminology eventually changed some, the implication remained that when women were "troublesome," particularly in the context of a medical practice, and no clear medical or organic etiology was found for their complaints, many older physicians still automatically placed the female patient in the category of "hysterical" or as having a "conversion disorder."

Throughout history, there have been several diseases that we as neurologists did not recognize as having an organic basis for the problem and subsequently were labeled as mental or psychiatric problems. Some neurological diseases that have seen a recent transition on how they are perceived within the last century are things like dystonia deformans progressive (also known as idiopathic torsion dystonia and dystonia musculorum deformans), a movement disorder which was initially deemed to be psychogenic in nature.[13] Another movement disorder known as Gilles de la Tourette, before it was embraced by neurologists and found to have the origin of the pathology within the dopamine system, was initially thought to be a psychiatric disorder of impulse control.[14] Some illnesses like schizophrenia still remain under the realm of psychiatry, although there are clear indications for an organic cause (too much dopamine).[15] I feel this is also the case for extending appropriate diagnosis to women, especially young women with PD. Since a lot of YOPD does not present with motor symptoms until years later—after depression, anxiety, sleep disorders, pain, constipation have wreaked havoc in their lives—many women thus suffer silently or in the wrong specialist's hands, going for years before receiving the right diagnosis. These individuals present with symptoms which do not conform neatly into a set of guidelines for diagnosis, exposing themselves to not just a misdiagnosis but also to being labeled as "crazy" or a "malingerer." Oftentimes, these women, instead of being referred to a neurologist or MDS, are referred to a psychiatrist due to their symptoms of depression or anxiety disorder. In my experience, they are then often given a diagnosis of bipolar disorder, conversion disorder, or fibromyalgia, which is chronic pain syndrome, delaying further diagnosis and proper medical treatment.

This scenario unfortunately occurs commonly among women and, in my experience, occurs more frequently in women of various ethnic groups, particularly that of Hispanic origin, in this country. This lag in diagnosis not only hinders appropriate treatment for those individuals who are initially placed in a category other than neurological illness or Parkinson's. Moreover, the initial misdiagnosis interferes with the overall understanding of disease etiology. If such practices continue to prevail in this country, we will miss out on an opportunity to advance the science of PD, especially given recent data which suggest that Hispanics carry twice the risk for developing Parkinson's disease compared to non-Hispanics. [16] This is even more profoundly significant considering that by the year 2020, Hispanics are projected to be the largest minority making up the majority of the population. [17]

Another important factor to consider as a reason for misdiagnosis in minorities is language and cultural barriers. Culture is a big part of who a person is, and it would be a mistake to treat or diagnose someone without first understanding this principle. I know about this from experience. For instance, among my fellow Hispanics, especially those who are immigrants (newly arrived to the country), it is anathema to tell a woman she has anxiety or depression. Sometimes certain stigmas bound in traditional beliefs are carried forward; therefore, it would be less likely to see a Hispanic woman presenting of their own accord with depression or other early non-motor PD symptoms. Unless a doctor asks specifically about these symptoms, and is vigilant, there is bound to be not only a delay in diagnosis and, therefore, a decreasing quality of life. The physician must inspire confidence and trust. Oftentimes, for example, Hispanics will only open up to other Hispanic professions, which may make diagnosis more difficult, since there is already a limited number of neurologists and movement disorder specialists, much less those who are Latino, and even less often, those who are Latino female doctors.

I suspect that other monitories like my own also feel more at ease in discussing their health issues with someone of their own cultural affiliation, and if such a doctor is not available, people may choose not to see a doctor at all. If they do choose to see a doctor outside their cultural affiliation, then there is the very real problem of misinterpretation, from the patient to the doctor, and vice versa.

It would serve the medical field well to keep an open mind, not disregarding the importance of understanding the cultural and language differences of their patients—when evaluating for a neurological condition, or any other medical illness, for that matter—also taking into account age, ethnicity, and gender. The one thing the science of medicine has taught me is that, although there are rules and guidelines by which we as physicians exercise our art, these are ever changing. This is best exemplified by an excerpt by author Thomas Szasz, who wrote: "[once] when religion was strong and science weak, men mistook magic for medicine; now when science is strong and religion is weak, men mistake medicine for magic."[18]

Even though we are taught to think in simple terms, of one disease explaining all symptoms in an individual, this is not 100% accurate for all individuals every single time. I should know; I am living proof of this. As I often say, just because I attended medical school and studied the textbooks, it does not mean that my body will conform to any given set of rules set forth within those books. I think this is why I have always been better than most at solving intricate and difficult cases because I have learned that someone will always come along to challenge all the rules in medicine, as in life.

Therefore, when dealing with Parkinson's disease, particularly of young onset or dealing with varying gender presentations, one must be careful to not oversimplify. We are all unique, complex individuals. In order to avoid misdiagnosis, we must learn to *listen* not just hear and to *see* not just look. The late Dr. John Calverley (1932-2004), a brilliant neurologist whom I had the honor of training under as a resident, said that "if you pay attention, patients will give you the diagnosis 90% of the time through a good history taking." Thus, as physicians, we have a responsibility to our patients to care for them and, above all, "do no harm," following the Hippocratic Oath. When we fail to consider alternatives, oversimplify, or dismiss someone's symptoms, we are essentially hurting our patients by omission. This kind of narrow-mindedness can be dangerous and counterproductive. If all physicians thought this way, the science of medicine would never advance!

We are individuals first and foremost, and the challenge for the medical community in regard to PD diagnosis and treatment is to assess the patients individually as well as within the scope of a larger picture, taking into account their backgrounds as well as what we have gleaned from others, including presentations, trials, and successes. This individualized focus is imperative considering the millions of people who are suffering from more than one malady!

This is particularly true in diagnosing YOPD; a misdiagnosis can have lifelong ramifications. We know early treatment and diagnosis can lead to a better quality of life. And in the case of young adults with PD, the preservation of quality of life is even more imperative in many ways; we want to see these young patients maintain an active role in society as a spouse, mother, caregiver, and professional. All of us—patients, physicians, loved ones, and caregivers—should maintain an open mind to effectively witness and treat this incurable disease.

I, too, was a victim of closed-minded thinking, assuming this or that about me, my mental status, my physical symptoms, and whether or not I was making up or imagining symptoms. My YOPD was eventually diagnosed accurately in 2008 after countless doctor visits, along with numerous tests which fell short of a brain biopsy. The whole ordeal was frustrating and infuriating. In fact, I was often infuriated at myself, thinking perhaps everyone was right and I indeed was imagining my symptoms. The blow to a young woman's self-esteem and willingness to trust her body and mind is devastating . . . and completely unnecessary.

An open mind, a listening heart, and a trained eye is the kind of specialist a woman with YOPD should expect and demand. I am fortunate to have found my wonderful doctor, friend, and colleague. She is truly a woman healer: Dr. Mya Schiess, professor and vice chair of the Department of Neurology at UT-Houston and director of the Movement Disorders Clinic & Fellowship.

I encourage everyone to continue to keep an open mind; once

in a while, when a young woman does not fit the mold, look beyond appearances. As it turns out, from all my research, I am a fairly typical female YOPD patient with presentation of pain (86% of all PD patients), fatigue (55% of PD patients), depression (one-third of PD patients can have this as initial symptom), constipation, bradykinesia, loss of smell, rest tremors (although mine are minimal), visual disturbances, rigidity, and signs and symptoms of dystonia.[19] If we are to become more effective at treating and diagnosing PD in women and enrolling patients in early trials, we must learn to think outside the box! To be able to increase our rate of accuracy in early PD diagnosis, not just in women but in all PD patients, surely having a biomarker will greatly improve our diagnostic accuracy; but in the meantime, we must serve as teaching tools for physicians to help each other recognize common and frequent symptoms found in women with PD, as above, which can actually present themselves years before the motor symptoms manifest themselves.[20] After all, having the right diagnosis is crucial for the success of any study, particularly one where you are looking at modifying the disease process. It's nearly impossible to find a cure or something to stop the progression if we don't even have the right disease—which has been the case in about fifty percent of those Parkinson's patients enrolled in early PD trials.[21]

5

Coping with Parkinson's: Spirituality, Religion & Health

"You must live your life from beginning to end; no one else can do it for you."

~ Hopi Proverb

Although it is not uncommon for people who initially receive the diagnosis of Parkinson's to feel like they have been given a "life sentence," or as if they had "the worst day" of their lives, the key to avoid getting stuck in this perpetual feeling and to continue to find meaning in life is to find a way to be empowered and to empower others with that same knowledge. We may not be able to change our circumstances, but we sure can do a lot about our own attitudes! You can either choose to panic in the face of a deteriorating illness with no cure, be paralyzed by the unknown, or embrace prayer and look for the greater good, thus empowering yourself and allowing healing to commence. This of course does not happen overnight for most of us; it is human nature, after all, to feel sorrow for our losses or our illnesses, especially when struck at a young age. We as Parkinson's patients, like any other person experiencing a chronic illness or suffering a traumatic loss, are not immune to experiencing the full gamut of emotions. We will often go through the five stages of grief: denial, bargaining, acceptance, anger, and depression.[1] And yes, these are out of typical order. I did this purposely because we as human beings have a tendency to cycle in and out of any and all stages before reaching acceptance and learning to embrace life once more. The important thing to remember is that PD is a lifelong process. Even when you have reached acceptance as the disease progresses, there may be dark days that make you question everything, get angry and upset all over again, as I have a time or two. There is no shame in this. Even our Lord Jesus got angry at unfair situations, but the key is not letting that anger consume you or take over your life. Rather, learn to acknowledge the emotions within, like fear, anger, and frustration, and then move on. Do not fuel them and drag them with you, allowing them to weigh you down. To be successful at living with a chronic progressive disease, you must let the unimportant things go and leave the rest in the hands of a higher power. This is where having faith is extremely important. Faith is *the substance of things hoped for, the evidence of things not seen.*[2] Our life should be lived as if a cure is already on the way!

Living with all of the idiosyncrasies of having Parkinson's disease can be too much for one person to bear at times. This is where trusting and leaning on someone else to help shoulder the burden can make a huge difference in an already stressful life. What better place to leave all of our stresses and fears than at the doorsteps of someone else wiser and more powerful than we are, like God. I love this concept because . . . what happens to things we leave behind at someone's door? We walk away and forget about them. Likewise, have you ever noticed that you might be looking for something, say your phone, all over the house and as soon as you step into another room you forget what it was you were looking for? Let me tell you, you are not alone. This type of forgetfulness happens to all of us. Our brains are wired this way. This phenomenon is known as the "door effect," which leads to forgetfulness. When you go from one room to another, you no longer can see what is in the other room, so your brain forgets. I believe this is our own brain's way of coping in order to be able to deal with painful traumatic experiences.[3, 4] I suggest that by doing this mental exercise metaphorically—leaving things at the door or imagining yourself walking through a door to a better place—you will be forcing your mind to file away the painful, negative memories and begin anew.

Another thing I have learned through my years of dealing with this illness as patient, physician, and caregiver is that it is okay to get angry or to cry until there are no more tears. This leads the way for a strong voice that is uniquely you to blossom. Holding back emotions, especially anger and frustration, is unhealthy on many levels. Eventually these emotions will rear their ugly heads one way or another, usually at the worst possible times, and are often directed toward loved ones who are only trying to help,

Everyone is different and needs different amounts of time to heal in the processing of a PD diagnosis and dealing with the reality that is Parkinson's. Eventually, we must all begin to heal; otherwise, we are at great risk of getting stuck for the rest of our lives and never moving forward. This would be a huge disservice to you and your loved ones. I once read that "delay is the deadliest form of denial."[5] We cannot make progress if we do not learn to adapt and realize that change is as much a part of life as being born and dying. We can't go around feeling sorry for ourselves; there are always worse things that can happen to us, I know. I have wept at the untimely death of a child with brain cancer and sat at the foot of the bed of many Parkinson's patients dying, after suffering for years, some of them ending up alone, causing me to wonder where their loved ones were at such a crucial time of need? But even for those patients who had family members and loved ones nearby, I still wept if their afterlife was uncertain, asking God for mercy on their souls . . . because for me, there is nothing more tragic than spending a lifetime suffering, only to continue suffering in an afterlife. Like Plato, I, too, feel that "the greatest mistake in treatment of diseases is that there are physicians for the body and physicians for the soul, although the two cannot be separated."[6] He thought that, just like one could not separate the eyes from the head, neither could one separate the soul from the body.[7]

My goal is to encourage PD treatment along with healing of patients as a whole, beliefs and all, and not just simply for the disease! As Wendell Reber wrote in the *Journal of the American Medical Association*: We can't forget that "we are such stuff as dreams are made of," because treating only the "outer casement of an individual," leads only to shortcomings and an unfulfilled person with PD.[8, 9]

For years, training of physicians did not include dealings outside of the physical realm. However, in recent years, I am proud to announce that certain medical schools have begun to develop programs emphasizing the need for treatment of the individual as a whole: body, mind, and soul as Plato once proposed. Today, more than one third of the nation's medical schools offer a course in faith and medicine.[10] This new direction of training future doctors makes perfect sense to me, given the fact that in ancient times, it was faith that brought about a cure. Christianity was the religion associated with healing. Christians transformed the world by reaching out to the suffering of the infirm, offering healing for their bodies and souls.[11] It was the Christian belief of charity based on love rather than mere "civic duty" that infused care of the sick with a spirituality underpinning.[12] So in fact, when first-century healers took care of patients, they did so as an imitation of Jesus' teachings.[13] Therefore, when someone prays at the bedside of a patient, they leave God with that patient.[14]

The positive effects of religion can be seen even outside the supernatural realm, extending into a person's social, physical, and psychological life. The findings reveal that those who are treated in this "whole" fashion (i.e., both mind and body) tend to do much better as compared to those that only receive care for their physical ailments. Spirituality and religion appear to play a big role in health, particularly for those who suffer from chronic illnesses, like Parkinson's disease.

Recently, a number of studies have "found increasing proof of the inseparability of body and mind."[15] One interesting aspect of neuroscience research is that repeated meditation or praying has shown to alter the brain structure in as little as eight weeks.[16] These changes are specific to areas of attention, learning, and mood regulation, all of which are impaired in Parkinson's.[17] This should really not be a surprise.

To most of us who exercise regularly, our muscles stretch and grow and become stronger the more we exercise them, as does the brain with persistent use and mental training. So let's get to praying and meditating on a regular basis, and let those neurons blossom into new connections.

The benefits of prayer, meditation, and religiosity result in the brain getting stronger. When viewed under a PET scan, the brain seems to "light up like a Christmas tree" during meditation, for example.[18] Many studies have suggested that medically ill older individuals, especially those who had depression, were quicker to recover from depression the more religious they were, compared to those who did not have religious beliefs.[19] This is particularly important in women with PD, but also in all Parkinson's patients, because depression is an intrinsic part of the illness. It is these negative feelings that impact our lives and shape our attitudes and color our perspectives in our daily living toward ourselves and others even more than the motor symptoms—to the point of potentially making us feel isolated and suicidal. So we must find a holistic way to combat our depression, sense of apathy, and anxiety in a positive fashion to enhance our lives as well as that of those around us. We can only accomplish this through a team approach by working with your physician to obtain proper medical treatments and by establishing a rapport with a group where the spirit can be fostered, like a Bible study group, for example.

According to data from a 2008 report, the American Religion Identification Survey (ARIS), in which US adults were questioned regarding the existence of God, 2.9% said there was no such thing; 4.3% stated there was no way to know; 5.7% were not certain; 12.1% claimed to believe in a higher power but did not believe in a personal God; 69.5% stated they believed in a personal God; and the rest refused to answer (6.1%). Although much of the work and research in this field has been carried out by those with interest in the Divine, their findings are still pertinent to a diverse group like women with Parkinson's disease.[20] Both the *Handbook of Religion and Health* and the Duke Center for Spirituality, Theology and Health[21, 22] confirmed that depressed patients were more likely than non-depressed individuals to have no religious affiliation and were less likely to attend church, pray, or read scripture, but the opposite was true for those that experienced a remission of their depression.[23] A combination of frequent religious attendance, prayer, and Bible study increased the speed of remission of depression.[24] Therefore, having a religious belief and actively practicing that belief not only improves your mood but does it faster. I, too, have had serious doubts about my life's purpose, possibly no longer being able to practice my art and chosen vocation. I have faced the bleak abyss of depression, desperation, and hopelessness at least once during my eight-year battle with this disease, caused by mental and physical fatigue but also brought on at least once by a medication reaction. The only thing, however, that kept me going and prevented me from giving up on myself aside from my daughter is the trust and faith I have in God. It is this faith that allows me to see that everything happens for a reason and, if I trust in Him, things will work out for the best, or even better than I could ever anticipate.

Furthermore, I believe that each one of us women with PD has unique talents that will help forge our own destinies, which can ultimately benefit others beyond ourselves. After all, as John Gardner once quipped, "When people are serving, life is no longer meaningless."[25] I have learned this from personal experience dealing with patients and families with PD: the more involved I have become in their lives, the greater the inner strength I have built, even as my body failed me. The satisfaction of helping someone in need is more than enough to overcome my own weaknesses. This is the same sentiment for all PD advocates I have ever encountered. It is those who unfortunately feel that they are alone or have nothing to give or share with one another that experience the greatest devastation and isolation when the waves of fear, anxiety, and depression come knocking at the door. Tragically, the end result can be something like what happened at the beginning of 2014 among several PD patients (mostly women) who had been battling PD for years and felt trapped with no way out. Sadly for these individuals, life had become meaningless, and the only relief they could find was suicide. Because we as women bear the brunt of the family issues and still have to be caregivers and spouses and have jobs, even when our bodies demand otherwise, the pressure can really build up. Therefore, it is imperative that everyone find a good support group to lean on. The best ones are the ones entirely made up of women in which you can interact personally, I believe, because it helps you discuss the salient issues that we all face on a daily basis plus gives the added bonus of socializing. But sometimes, it is not possible to make these support groups either, because there are none in our area or because our life circumstances prohibit us from going out or joining these groups. Fortunately, in the age of social media, you can connect with anyone you want around the globe. There are many online support groups. Some are local, while others are global. The best way to find these is by asking other people with Parkinson's or the larger Parkinson's foundations to direct you. Some of these sites have forums where you can ask questions from experts or other patients. I have met wonderful people from around the world via these forums, some of whom I have gotten to later meet in person at PD events. So, you should not feel alone in this . . . because you are not! Even if you don't have a computer, the national foundations have hotlines to help point you in the right direction and connect you to groups, even if you happen to live outside of the US.

So, I say to you, my esteemed reader: don't lose hope, hang on to your faith, be open-minded, and be open to change. Welcome change like the seasons, for it is a part of life.

Another reason to keep the faith is not only to ward off negative feelings but to combat the emotional fatigue that comes from getting involved with people and causes. Sometimes we become so invested in people, in human relations that we can become stressed and short-tempered, such as in the case of my family, especially with my dad's battle with cancer over the past year. You can become so emotionally fragile and spent. Add to the mix your illness along with all of your duties of mother, wife, daughter, friend, etc., and your body is like a tight guitar string ready to break at the slightest pluck. Under such enormous stress, your brain consumes dopamine at a rate that cannot easily be replaced and maintained, leaving you not only mentally and physically exhausted but feeling like your Parkinson's symptoms just went into overdrive! This roller coaster of emotions can make anyone, even the sanest of individuals, feel schizophrenic at times. Although you may think you are not stressed or getting depressed, you may wonder why you are not eating as before, or sleeping as before, or worse, why tiny drops of fluid seem to come rolling down your cheeks at the most inopportune times, making you feel like you have even less control over your body, causing greater frustration and discontentment.

I have interviewed many patients in my day, watching their eyes fill up with tears, followed by a resounding denial of being depressed. Perhaps some of these women were right; they were NOT depressed but simply overwhelmed, exhausted. Finding themselves at their wits' end, what they needed most was a friend, someone to listen, a sympathetic ear. Sure, they may have also required antidepressants or anti-anxiety medications, but more than anything else they needed spiritual healing, someone to pray over them, to say, "It's going to be okay. You are not alone. It will get better. Don't lose hope."

We have all heard that hope is the last to die. A person can live without food for a couple of weeks, without water a few days, without oxygen a few minutes . . . but without hope we cannot live a single second!

For those of us with chronic illnesses, having faith along with regular church attendance helps to increase one's life expectancy by at least eight years on average.[26] I firmly believe this is one of the main reasons why a powerful man of God like Reverend Billy Graham continues to thrive at ninety-plus years of age, still writing books and continuing to preach even after twenty-plus years of dealing with PD. Who would have thought that, when we first met at a church revival at Rice University, standing there beside him at my young age of thirteen, we would end up sharing not just God but Parkinson's disease as well?

Having faith and religion allows people better coping skills too, giving them reduced anxiety, especially about death, and helping to put in perspective their own illnesses, finding meaning in them, dealing with their own mortality. Finally, it allows people to move forward to a Plan B, by giving emotional comfort and resilience as they learn to embrace their new lives. What is most interesting is that it appears to be most helpful for certain groups, such as women, the elderly, and African

Americans. Remember, women are usually the caregivers, ones who help raise grandchildren, oftentimes taking care of ill parents along with children and spouses, even when they themselves are ill. So yes, we need this extra coping mechanism—having a faith—to be able to juggle all our responsibilities and duties, particularly when we are stuck in a low-income situation or find ourselves without spousal support for reasons of divorce or death, etc.

To emphasize the role of and importance of developing a spiritual side as a person or woman with PD in the treatment of this disease is a study of coping mechanisms for various neurological diseases. In this study, it was of note that those who had Parkinson scored the highest in "religious relief" and a "quest for sense."[27] Unlike other neurological patients, those with Parkinson's tend to maintain their faith in spite of the severity of the disease. This is great news. We do not lose hope easily! We know that, as Parkinson's patients, we are strong, and as women, we are fearless. Imagine what we can accomplish if we just put our minds to it!

So then, what will my legacy be? What about yours? Will it be one of victory or one of defeat?

Your Parkinson's does not have to define you or make you a prisoner with a life sentence. You always have a say in your life. Your circumstances may not be able to change, but your outlook on life and your attitude can be modified. You can be empowered to pray for yourself and others by a simple choice; you can alter your path and your destiny and become the woman you always wanted to be by achieving spiritual wellbeing, meaning a sense *"of good health as a whole person and as unique woman,"* who happens to have PD.[28]

The best way to be empowered is to write your own survival story, according to experts in the field of dealing with women who have severe emotional, physical, and health disabilities from chronic, progressive incurable illnesses. One such expert is a close friend of mine, Wilma, who says that women who write their stories have a higher sense of belonging, connection, and are able to overcome the devastation of adversities thrust upon them.[29] Don't be afraid to write your story. No one *but you* is the expert on *you* and what you are feeling, the path you have walked. Remember, let it come from deep within you, understanding who you are on many levels: cultural, religious, spiritual, family upbringing, as well as how you view your place in the world. You must look beyond the present "in general" and instead look at all the small battles you have already won that got you where you are today. Keep writing until you feel hope surge anew in your life. My recommendations are to discuss with your doctor any spiritual concerns you might have.[30]

- DO spend some time thinking about religious and spiritual questions.
- DON'T be afraid to tackle the big issues in your life. Healing always comes from within.
- DO let yourself (or your loved one who has PD) talk about spirituality or religion. These things may help influence both your mental and health outcomes in the long run, thrusting you forward to a greater destiny and happier you.

The benefits are extremely worth your while:
- Faster recovery from illness or any personal loss, such as the death of a loved one.
- Improvement in your confidence and self-esteem, which makes you more attractive.
- Better relationships.
- Increase in creativity and in values, such as patience, kindness, hope, honesty, love, joy, wisdom.
- Inner peace and ease of acceptance of our difficult situations, helping to make sense of them as well.

I like to think of our spiritual journey with PD as a beautification process. Being a PD Diva, I love fine china. Even as a child, I loved playing with dainty tea sets. I enjoyed having them so much that, over the years; I have accumulated a good number of tea sets. When my daughter was born, I was ecstatic to be able to pass on my collection on to her. I wanted for her to enjoy them as much as I had. And she did! When she was just a toddler, because some of the sets are miniature, she and I would play tea party with these. She absolutely loved playing with them, which of course brought me much joy. Being so young, a few pieces got damaged, but this was worth the price for the memories we made together. Therefore, when I envision a piece of fine china, I think of a pristine porcelain cup that is intricately decorated with painstaking detail in bold, beautiful colors by a master artisan, or the tea set my grandmother bequeathed me. I had loved that set since the day my grandfather bought it for her, not just for its beauty but because the teapot also played a piece by Mozart—enjoy some tea while soothing your senses and spirit!

We are just like this unique tea set. Like us, the tea set was once just a lump of clay. It, like us at times, perhaps even before our disease, was content to be a pile of clay because its potential and limits had never been stretched. Many of us before Parkinson's came into our lives were content being who we were, thinking what we had was enough. Some of us thought life could not get any better. Yet, as the artisan saw greater potential in the tea set, we too have great potential that can only be brought out through molding, shaping, and heating in the hot furnace of life, i.e., living with PD.

Although the journey with PD can be uncomfortable at best and undesirable at worst, we can learn to endure the process. After all, I survived cancer when I was told I had only a few months to live. And every time we think we have the hang of it, a new test or challenge comes our way in the form of new symptoms or side effect, which we must once again learn to endure. And we can!

When we look at our own reflections in the mirror, we can be proud of our transformation from a simple lump of clay to a masterpiece and true work of art—a transformation that could only have been accomplished along this Parkinson's journey.

Someday, all of us beautiful teacups will adorn the table of the Master Artisan in Heaven when our journey here is complete.

6

Raising Children When Mom has Parkinson's

"Without injury and irritation the oyster will not produce a pearl."
~ *Elizabeth George*

I have often said that becoming a neurologist was infinitesimally easier than raising kids. Even in the toughest crises of life and death situations, I often felt much more at ease dealing with some of the complex issues of medicine/neurology than being a mom.

After all, I spent twelve years training to become a neurologist but only seven months to have my tiny, four-pound baby girl, for which a manual was not even included. Even though my husband and I were both physicians, we still had to undergo CPR training to care for this preemie beautiful child before we could take her home. Medical training we had plenty, but no experience as parents! Yet like everyone else, we had to learn what made her special and unique.

Those of you who have children know from experience that as soon as you figure something out, there is a new challenge or new stage, and you have to move on and start the learning process all over again. As moms with PD, we have to learn to fly from the seat of our pants. Although our bodies may not always be the fastest, our minds make up for it in creativity, finding ways to work around our unique disease. My daughter learned this from a very young age, especially since she was so young when I got diagnosed. At one point, I was almost completely dependent on others for transportation, running errands, etc. Just getting around required me to use various walking assistive devices. Yet despite my lack of mobility, my daughter knew that although my body was slow, my mind was not. She told her dad once, "Mom's brain is fast." She knew I was still involved in her life, and I was not going to miss much of what was important to her. This was very comforting to her because all children need rules, consistency, and tons of love.

Having a chronic illness like Parkinson's, in which your life is in constant flux both mentally and physically, can wreak havoc on anyone. Then throw in the mix having to raise another human being who is completely and solely dependent on you for all his/her needs, when most days you can't even take care of yourself. Makes for a very interesting life, to say the least! It helps a lot if you have a loving, caring partner who is devoted and involved not just in your care but also in the care of the children. However, this may be a fantasy world for some parents out there, who not only have to worry about managing their own disease, but also solely providing for a child. You would have to be a magician to be able to juggle everything. Just thinking about it wears me out!

I think I need a nap.

But as more and more people like me and you (WE!) are diagnosed with young onset Parkinson's disease or even typical PD (since some of us are waiting longer to have children), this issue of how to raise children in the midst of Parkinson's becomes an extremely crucial one!

At the onset of symptoms and after initial diagnosis, once the shock has worn off, it is not uncommon to begin to ask a million questions.

- Will I be around to see my child grow up?
- Will I be able to partake in their daily and social activities?
- Will I be able to have (more) children?
- How do I tell my child I have PD?
- Should I tell?

Oh, the list is long, and these are just a few of the many questions your brain will conjure up. But let's address these for starters.

Will I be around . . . ?

First, chances are good that you will be able to see your child grow up since, according to current medical thinking, Parkinson's disease does not necessarily shorten life span, although it is the fourteenth leading cause of death. Particularly for those who start PD treatment early and are followed by a movement disorder specialist or neurologist have a greater chance for a better quality of life.[1]

Can I partake in activities . . . ?

Although at present there is no cure for PD, there are a myriad of treatment options, including medications, surgical procedures, and holistic methods, like exercising (cycling, yoga, swimming, etc.), art therapy, dancing (tango, etc.), which may not only improve motor function and but also improve vitality and flexibility—a game winner when it comes to caring for your little ones.

Should I tell . . . ?

Honesty is the best policy. You should tell them. Arm them with age-appropriate information and resources.

There is no time like the present time. Children are very perceptive and know when something is going on even when you don't say anything. There are many books available to help guide your conversation. If at all possible, sit down to talk to your children as a family. This will reassure them and reinforce their feeling of security that things at home will continue as they have been, or as close to it as possible.

Reach out to professionals, online sites, and books that can help guide conversation with your loved ones, whether they are three, teenage, or even adult age.

I was diagnosed with Parkinson's when my daughter was six years old. Before then, my grandmother, who also had PD, lived with us. My child has practically grown up with Parkinson's since she was a toddler due to my profession as well as having been around her great-grandmother. Yet, when I was diagnosed, we still sat down and talked about it, particularly to dispel her concern that I would not be around to see her grow up, since my grandmother who had battled with PD over fifteen years, died six months after coming to live with us.

It was normal in our home to help and care for those with this illness; after my grandmother's diagnosis, followed by mine, Parkinson's took center stage in all of our personal lives. After she passed away and I developed symptoms of Parkinson's a year and a half later, my daughter became very anxious and worried that I might die as well. This is where consistency helped tremendously and continues to do so to this day. I have reassured her that grandma's death was due to her being very elderly and having a brain tumor, not due to PD. Although it was true that she lived with PD for a long time and caused her to be sicker in the end due to her underlying condition, it was not the PD that killed her. Despite my family history, my Parkinson's was not going to affect how long I lived; people with PD live normal life spans. Also I have reinforced to my daughter that fortunately now there are so many new medicines that can make people have nearly normal lives for a long time, as well as medicines that were not available when grandma got sick.

Now that my daughter is a teenager, she occasionally worries if *she* will get PD. I have told her that Parkinson's or *'parkinspins'* as we like to call it, is NOT usually a hereditary disease (less than 10%). Nevertheless, because grandma had it and I have it, she has a higher chance of getting this disease as do her children. However, I STRESS to her that this is the reason I work as a research advocate with PDF and other organizations, like the Muhammad Ali Parkinson's Center. Even though I can no longer work as a neurologist and be a Parkinson's doctor, I can still have an impact on PD by helping people with Parkinson's everywhere. My job now is to aid in steering research toward finding a cure, so that my daughter and others like her will not have to live with this disease! This brings her a lot of comfort because she trusts me as a mom and has seen me care for my patients as a doctor over the years.

Here are a few things that I have learned as a parent with PD, dealing with my own daily personal battle with this illness. Perhaps, some of my insights might be of use to those of you who have children or grandchildren living with you.

- The first thing, never underestimate your children's intelligence no matter their age. They may not understand everything, but they are smarter than you think, and they will always take cues from you as to what is going on. If you are not upfront and explain to them, at a level appropriate to their age, they will be potentially traumatized, forever worried about you. This can lead to acting out, depression, anxiety, clinginess, and even overprotectiveness toward you, leading toward separation anxiety in the very young. They may also develop night terrors or nightmares. They may become withdrawn or aggressive.

  Act out your symptoms with them; make it a game if they are, say, under age seven. Talk about the "wiggles" or the "shakes," or being taken over by a "slow" bug. Tell them that, with their assistance some of these symptoms can get better—for example, you can walk faster if they hold your hand. Get them involved in your Parkinson's projects or any other projects. My daughter's Girl Scout troop planted tulips one year to raise awareness in our community. Another time, my daughter made bracelets for me to distribute at one of my PD talks, again to raise awareness. **Empower them.**

- Initially, since my daughter was only three when my grandmother died, when I got diagnosed with PD, she became extremely upset each time I left the house. She was afraid of me dying, because all she knew was that 'grandma was sick with Parkinson's, could not walk, and subsequently went to heaven. So when she overheard me talking to my husband after returning from my Houston visit to my neurologist, which confirmed the diagnosis, before I had a chance to sit down with her and realize what her mind had processed, she assumed I would be dying soon as well and began to have separation anxiety.

I had to explain that grandma died because she had cancer, was elderly and missed grandpa already in heaven so went to be with him, not because of the Parkinson's; 'mommy' on the other hand would be around a very LONG time-even until she went to college and got married. Although, I explained I might get shakier and slower too like grandma. Reminded her about how grandma was still a hoot and fun to do things with like paint even when she was sick! And how much we still loved her and she loved us.

I also explained that because I was getting this "grandma disease," I needed a little vacation from work to get better (because closing my office and no longer being around my employees who were like family to us also disturbed her). If I no longer had to work and spend all my time with my patients, I could instead spend ALL my time with her doing "mommy things" (i.e., fun things). This idea she immediately embraced and asked that I not return to work until she went to college! (She is still holding me to this, even though she is a teenager!)

I further explained that I would need her help from time to time because sometimes, I might just be too slow to get dressed or too shaky to do her hair or carry her or put her shoes on. However, this did not mean I did not love her or want to do things for her and with her. I deputized her as Mommy's Little Helper, which made her happy. Now she had a role . . . and a mission. **Reassure them.**

• Encourage whatever creativity they might express with regard to helping with your symptoms. My daughter wanted to help me raise awareness for Parkinson's, so she drew a tulip, stating: "I am not shaky, I am dancing!"

Even now as she has gotten older and is no longer a toddler, we still have special mom and daughter times. She also knows that I may be somewhat SLOW in my feet (walking, moving) but FAST in my HEAD, although I often have trouble keeping up with her musical beats and rhythms. Yet, we still sing, dance and make music together! **Let them dance.**

- Encourage spirituality as well. Use your illness to teach your children values. Your children will learn courage, love, and compassion and develop integrity and character by the way you show love and compassion to others and handle adversity. I often tell my daughter that our life is defined not by what obstacles and challenges come our way but how we handle them. I remind her always about the importance of having a dream, even when we become a hundred years old, disabled, or chronically ill. The key is to foster hope in our children. My daughter likes two stories that I share with her. The first is concerning Walt Disney, who was rejected by three hundred two banks before he finally got a "yes" and was approved for a loan to build his dream: the Disney Empire.[2]

   The second story is borrowed in part from one of her grandfather's favorite boxers, who also happens to be battling Parkinson's disease—the former boxing champion, Muhammad Ali. After all, as Ali would say, "champions are not made in the gym (or in school, etc.), they are made from what they have deep within their heart, a drive, a vision, a desire" to make things better for yourself and others.[3] Give them hope.

- The most important thing in raising children when you have a chronic illness like PD is to maintain a sense of normalcy as much as possible in their lives. Your problems should not be their problems. They already worry enough. Oh, and be sure to remind them that PD is NOT contagious and just because you have it DOES NOT mean they will too. Let them be children. Allow them to participate in activities in and out of school, have friends over, and *play play play*. Teach them new things, help them with their homework, spend free time with them, show them unconditional love, and find games that both you and they can enjoy. For example, a board game, coloring/drawing, guessing games (especially funny if your voice is off, or if you are dyskinetic or having bad tremors), dominoes, or cards (especially if you use cookies as winnings). Play Wii together, especially Brain Academy (or a similar game on Nintendo DS) as well as balance games; not only will you have loads of fun as you struggle and make complete fools of yourselves, but you will also be enhancing your brain cell connections and improving your PD symptoms. If you're having a really good day, go for a walk with your children, ride bikes together (especially in tandem), or go for a swim. All of these activities will not only help you bond with your child, but will help your PD as well. **Give them normalcy.**

- Laugh at your symptoms and clumsiness together, not in a mean way, but because, well, sometimes it really *is* funny! For example, there was the time my family went to eat Japanese food, and I could not use my chopsticks very well. I kept accidentally flinging sushi across the table a la Julia Roberts, and when we got in the car, I noticed that my pants were nicely decorated with rice. We all had a big laugh about this on the way home. Ask your children to show you how they see you, and then ask them to tell you how they feel about you. You'll be amazed at what you might discover in those brains of theirs! After all, laughter is the best medicine. My daughter thinks of me as a silly, crazy, fun, smart, wild-haired mom who sometimes just can't get it right. I love that. **Laugh with them.**

- Try to make their favorite foods when you are able to. Ask for their help only if absolutely necessary (you don't want to rob them of their childhood and force them to become your caregiver. It is not their role, and shouldn't be! You are still the parent, and they need to be children. Allow them to cook with you if they want to; they will enjoy making a mess with you if you are having a bad day with your PD. They will learn important things from you when you are having a good day. Either way, you will be building their self-esteem as you focus on their worlds. **Pamper them.**

• Remember, children are little sponges; they absorb everything and learn by example! Do try not to complain or be "ill" in front of them too much, because children are great emulators. The younger they are and less able to understand, they will begin to subconsciously "act" like you because they love you and identify with you. You don't want them to turn into hypochondriacs. They may start saying that their muscles are "stiff" or "tight" or become worried about having or developing tremors. Try to explain this is NOT contagious or hereditary. Validate their concerns to a certain point but be aware that this does not become an attention seeking behavior. If this is the case, you need to consult with a professional ASAP. Let them know it is not their responsibility to be your caregiver. You are still the one that will care for them. Their only job is to be children, be happy. Reassure them and let them know that **PD or no PD, they are number one**!

Will I be able to have (more) children . . . ?
Fertility, as far as we know, is not altered due to Parkinson's, but there really is no definitive information. What we know as of now is limited, but my observations are that fertility is not impaired and that women with PD are able to conceive and have children. However, as I mentioned in the chapter on pregnancy and PD, this is not without consequences. Thus, you must talk to your physician at length and determine the best plan of action for you as an individual. Also keep in mind that some PD women may also have other comorbidities, the treatments for which may come into play when deciding on whether or not to conceive. After all,

PD does not exist in a vacuum. Other personal factors must come into the decision-making process as well.

Remember, our children are our greatest assets, so cherish them always. They can be your greatest source of encouragement, strength, and reason for carrying on the good fight, even when the going gets tough. When my daughter was younger, and I was much more incapacitated than I am today, it was her love and daily songs that would keep me going. Whatever the day's events—good, bad, or funny—she would rhyme and sing for me.

My daughter also loved for me to sing to her before bedtime, of course, because it was soothing to her as a young child, but now she likes me to sing to her because it is funny. My once melodious voice has turned into a veritable croak due to my PD and dystonia of my vocal cords (dysphonia), and my laughter is more like an old hag's cackle. She even made several recordings of me to keep with her and thinks that my new talents might land me on the steps of Hollywood to play all the evil villains' voices. Despite the barks and obvious misses in pitch and rhythm, she still loves to hear me sing and laugh. Although, once in a while, she will poke me at church while we are singing . . . I hope God does not mind my voice too much. Interestingly enough, if I sing in Spanish or another language, the vocal dysphonia is not as severe.

So, I thank Parkinson's disease for allowing me to fully experience motherhood in a way that would not have been possible had I continued working full speed with my career as a neurologist and never had the bittersweet encounter with PD. I may not always have a lot of energy or be able to do all the things I wish I could do. Sometimes I have to rest all day just to be able to attend my daughter's extracurricular performances, but oh . . . it is worth it to see my daughter happy, knowing she is cherished.

I do have to admit that my culinary skills have improved greatly, and my family notices, since I have to add more color, spices, and textures to my food to compensate for my loss of smell, another PD symptom of mine. Whenever we get the chance, my daughter and I bake together. She likes for us to try different pie recipes. When we bake, we typically like to wear matching aprons: DIVA for me and DIVA IN TRAINING for her. Once we baked a Scandinavian dessert called "fattigmann," a fried pastry not unlike Mexican "sopapillas." We both ended up looking like we had been personally hand-dipped into the flour and sugar mix, which of course, just made us laugh hysterically.

From author and mother who has YOPD, Adele Pfrimmer Hensley: "When Clark was four years old, I painted all the children in his preschool class with clown faces. I was slow, but I completed the face painting. I realized that was the last time I would be able to volunteer in that way. Parkinson's disease has made me much less capable as a mom than I otherwise might have been. Conversely, it has given me a son who is much more compassionate than he might have been. He has had to step in and help when I could not. Parkinson's often gives a person a facial mask, but it does not let a person put up a false front of efficiency. Not even when that person is a mother."

7

Pregnancy and PD: What to Expect
When You Are Expecting

*"The best part of being pregnant...? You
don't have to suck in your gut."*

~ pregnancyhumor.com

First, you must get through pregnancy with PD, and that's no easy feat
. . . to enjoy motherhood in the midst of PD. Additionally, symptoms
of Parkinson's may worsen not just physically but emotionally during
pregnancy.[1] Furthermore, not all medications are safe to use during
pregnancy, which may leave you high and dry dealing with ten months
(yes, ten! . . . doctors always talk about nine months of pregnancy but they
try to sneak in that extra month thinking that since you are pregnant, you
won't notice) of pregnancy aches and pains plus the possible worsening of
PD symptoms, like tremors and depression. Even though pregnancy has
its own benefits, like eating whatever you want because you are "eating
for two," it can be ultra-stressful when combined with a chronic illness.
Therefore, it is not to be entered into lightly.

As more young women with early onset PD become pregnant, the
importance of knowing what to expect is crucial. Unfortunately, there
is very little information on the subject. It is my personal observation
working with various Parkinson's support groups through social media,
the cluster of women with YOPD appears to be localized in the West

Coast and Southwest here in the US. Australia also seems to have a large number of YOPD women active on social media PD support groups. But there is no epidemiological data to confirm the numbers of YOPD women and how to track their experiences. This is why a national PD registry, which includes pregnancy, is badly needed if we are to fully understand the nuances of pregnancy in women with YOPD. Although California has a PD registry, it does not cover pregnancy. Nebraska is the only state with a PD registry that includes pregnancy data.[2, 3] In May 2015, the state of Utah launched a PD registry to include all patients with Parkinson's and other movement disorders, and it will be linked to a cancer database in hopes of gathering statistics and genetic information; however, Utah does not have a Parkinson's pregnancy registry specifically.

I will try to summarize what we do know to date. Although data is scarce, it appears fertility is not impaired in Parkinson's disease.[4] However, because a large number of women diagnosed before age fifty are still menstruating, there is an impact on menstrual cycles.[5, 6]

Due to the limitations of data available on the topic of pregnancies in women with Parkinson's disease, we must look at this issue two-fold:

- Impact of Pregnancy on Parkinson's
- Effect Parkinson's has on Pregnancy

The role estrogen plays on PD is conflicting to say the least, according to the experts. The opinions as to whether estrogen is beneficial or detrimental is all over the spectrum—yes, estrogen helped symptoms; eh, it made no difference; no, estrogen made things worse. As I've mentioned, estrogen does seem to provide a protective role for the brain against certain neurological illnesses, like stroke and even PD. According to a small study looking at Parkinson's women and the issue of fertility, it was discovered that there was an apparent delay in PD in women with a higher number of pregnancies; these women had a longer fertile life.[7] This speaks volumes to me about the protective role of estrogen in women.

The Impact of Pregnancy on Parkinson's

There appears to be an increase in both motor and non-motor symptoms of PD during pregnancy. In my capacity as a research advocate, I have had the privilege to interact and work closely with many young women who have become pregnant. They have described to me a worsening of their PD symptoms during their pregnancy. However, most were more specific in stating that their symptoms usually got worse after the second trimester with only a few of them getting worse from the onset of the pregnancy. These women gave birth to full-term, healthy babies. Furthermore, several of them have continued to have children, despite their diagnosis of Parkinson's.

The take-home for this information is that, yes, PD symptoms seem to worsen during pregnancy but are transitory since they go back to baseline after delivery. PD does not appear to affect fertility or affect the fetus adversely, since most of these women were not on PD medications while they were pregnant. For those few women who had multiple childbirths although they carried a diagnosis of PD for five to eight years, the disease did not seem to have progressed very much since these women were still on relatively small doses of dopamine agonists or dopa replacement. It seems to me that given these anecdotal cases, having children might serve as a protective role even after the disease sets in. However, we do not have any current data to support this speculation at this time.

What we do know is that in a small study of thirty-six PD pregnancies, twenty-seven of them had either worsening or appearance of new symptoms of PD during or shortly after delivery.[8] This study partly confirms my observations. Only one report in the literature gives evidence of a new-onset occurrence of Parkinsonism (Parkinson's-like symptoms) at eleven weeks gestation. The disease resolved spontaneously after delivery.[9] This confirms once again what I have observed; pointing to estrogen's role of protection on the brain once the levels return to baseline. Obviously, more research is needed in this area still.

We still don't know much about the impact of Parkinson's medications on birth control pills or other anti-contraceptives, so if you do not want to get pregnant, I would recommend using double protection, like condoms combined with birth control pills. I highly recommend discussing this and all related issues with your physician prior to making any changes to your medical regimen or attempting conception.

The Effect Parkinson's on Pregnancy

The number one concern for all Parkinson's women who might suddenly become pregnant is the risk of birth defects caused from the intake of Parkinson's medications.[10] The other challenges are caring for a baby after birth, when you, the mom, has PD, as well as knowing which medications are safe to use while breastfeeding. Although I have provided a list as to which medications are considered relatively safe for breastfeeding, the problem is they block milk production, making it impossible to feed. Amantadine is the only medication shown to have caused heart defects in newborns with first trimester exposure. Often women are not even aware they are pregnant until well into their first trimester, during which time amantadine could cause serious repercussions.[11]

Restless Leg Syndrome (RLS), also known as Ekbom syndrome, is the most common movement disorder of pregnancy.[12] RLS is described as creepy-crawly sensations or actual restlessness in the legs with an irresistible need to move, usually only alleviated by walking. Symptoms can also occur in the arms, although less often and usually after treatment. [13] Since RLS is also a common symptom of Parkinson's, which might be exacerbated during pregnancy, we can expect Parkinson's women who get pregnant to experience these symptoms in some shape or form. RLS typically occurs during the second and third trimester, making it hard to differentiate between exacerbation of PD symptoms and garden-variety RLS due to pregnancy. RLS due to pregnancy resolves after delivery. One of the reasons it worsens in pregnancy is anemia, either from iron deficiency or folate deficiency, but can also be due to B12 deficiency, which is very common in Parkinson's disease.[14] Because of the association of RLS with the above deficiencies, if you or your loved one is symptomatic, you should have these vitamin levels tested, along with your iron levels. If any such deficiency is found, replacement is recommended, which typically will ameliorate symptoms. However, if low levels are not found, then replacement safety and utility are not yet ascertained.[15] In those cases, RLS should be treated symptomatically with dopamine agonists or dopamine replacement.

The main problem with RLS therapy is "augmentation," meaning an increasing need to escalate medication in order to control symptoms—plus, it tends to spread to other body parts, or symptoms begin to present during the day and not just at night. Typically dopamine agonists are used as the first line of treatment due to lower risk of augmentation compared to other dopaminergic compounds like levodopa.[16] However, in RLS of pregnancy and in PD patients who have RLS while pregnant, levodopa is the first-choice medication for those with enough symptoms requiring treatment, because compared to the dopamine agonists, L-dopa has a higher efficacy and safety profile in pregnancy. Pergolide (no longer available in the US) and Requip (ropinerole) have been associated with intrauterine growth retardation, digit malformation, and fetal deaths in animals.[17]

More women are now waiting longer to have children, putting themselves at that cusp between YOPD and typical PD. Combine that with the fact that recommendations for DBS treatment are now moving toward an earlier phase in the spectrum of PD, and these trends will bring about more discussions concerning pregnancy and DBS in the near future.[18] However, to date, the information available regarding DBS in pregnancy is very limited, particularly regarding safety of this procedure during pregnancy. So far, the only data available regarding safety in pregnancy comes from a three-case report of this DBS during pregnancy, conducted for treatment of dystonia. These three patients reportedly had successful pregnancies.[19, 20] Currently, since DBS is primarily employed after medications have failed, were not well tolerated, and/or were not producing the needed effect or causing dyskinesias in this chronically progressive disease, it is still reasonable to withhold the procedure until the postpartum period ensues to minimize risk to fetus. However, as the number of women with YOPD increases and the recommendations are now changing towards earlier DBS treatment, further in-depth studies will be necessary to thoroughly assess the potential benefits to the mother versus risks to the fetus.

Below I have provided you with a list of PD meds and their FDA categories as they apply to pregnancy. Nevertheless, you must review and discuss all of your options with your doctor thoroughly before thinking about getting pregnant, during pregnancy, during the postpartum period, and if you are planning on breastfeeding.

Drug	FDA Pregnancy Category	Breast-Feeding
levodopa	C	Do not use-no
data on milk		
rotigotine	C	No human data
amantadine	C	Do not use
trihexyphenidyl	C	No data on
excretion (milk)		
pramipexole	C	Do not use
ropinirole	C	Do not use
excreted in breast milk		
apomorphine	C	Can be used in preganancy, but no known studies available regarding transmission in breast milk
procyclidine	C	No data available

(21) According to US Food and Drug Administration, Assigned Pregnancy Categories as used in drug formularies. In this case, *Category C* means that animal reproduction studies have revealed an adverse effect on the fetus, and there are no adequate and well-controlled studies in humans, but potential benefits may warrant use of the drugs in pregnant women despite risks.

8

Love and Marriage in PD (Till Death Do Us Part)

"To love someone deeply gives you strength.
Being loved by someone deeply gives you courage."

~ Lao Tzu

In an age where love and marriage seem to be on the decline, how do we survive a marriage while living with a chronic, progressive, neurodegenerative illness?

Not an easy task, I tell you! It takes a lot of give and take from both parties, plus a whole lot of overlooking each other's faults, to have a happy and successful marriage. While divorce rates are on the rise, it is said that 50% of first marriages, 65% of second marriages, and 70% of third marriages end in divorce.[1] So in this case, practice does not make perfect, it seems. So if you are lucky enough to still be with your first mate, stick to it!

Not long ago, I heard someone say that young people are choosing to forgo marriage altogether or wait until they are in their late thirties or even early forties to wed, given the high divorce statistics in this country. Long gone are the days of sixty-plus-year wedding anniversaries like my grandparents had, who were married for sixty-eight years—the year they both passed away, six months apart.

Given the gravity of the situation in our society, I ponder how others with various neurological diseases are faring. Not a lot of data is available for Parkinson's patients regarding divorce, but from personal observation, it is more frequent than any of those, including myself, suffering or living with the illness would like it to be. However, I came across an article regarding another neurological group whose patients had severe, chronic, debilitating neurological deficits, such as spinal cord injuries and multiple sclerosis. We as PD patients have a lot in common with these groups of patients—progression of disease, chronic fatigue, bladder and sexual problems, etc. According to the article, those who suffered from these illnesses had twice the divorce rate than the regular population in the US, which is already astronomical.[2, 3] Moreover, it was more common among female patients.[4] In 1994, 20.7% of disabled adults were divorced, compared to 13.1% of non-disabled adults, and disabled individuals often had to go at it alone.[5] This got me thinking about the Parkinson's friends, patients, and colleagues I have come in contact with over the years; many faces and names bombarded my mind, immediately confirming this very notion of an ever-increasing number of divorces amongst my patients and friends who have been given chronic illnesses. So, I wondered what we could do as PD patients, family members, and carepartners to avoid going down this slippery road which leads to divorce.

Make no mistake: marriage is hard work especially the first seven years until you get comfortable with yourself and the role you are in. There is always that initial fear of being judged if we allow our personalities to come out full-blown. Now add a chronic illness diagnosis to this new setting of insecurity on both parts, and we are poised for disaster unless we have the right tools. Perhaps, my experiences in the subject will help some of you find the right tools and make the right choices for your lives.

We know that women respond to stress differently than men, as mentioned previously. It stands to reason that we would respond to treatment in an entirely different manner, independent of our physiologies. Don't forget for a second that we as women are viewed or valued the same by society as our male counterparts. It is expected of us to be able to multitask without breaking a sweat. Even though gender roles are changing in our society, we still tend to feel sorry or give more credit to a father who is alone working and rearing his children than we do women. It is almost expected that we are somehow super women. Whatever the educational or professional status, most women feel the need to "be in charge" of the family daily goings-on, the home, the children, the parents, the chores, and so on. Multitasking is nothing new for most of us (that's why some scientists believe women have a ticker corpus callosum (nerve bundle connecting both hemispheres). That's just a myth, but comparing brain sizes, women do have more gray matter (thinking neurons) than our male counterparts. Coincidence? I think not![6] But what happens when the woman is the one who becomes ill? Do the obligations suddenly banish or do they intensify? How does one cope?

Too frequently, PD women find themselves alone (with children and other responsibilities) as they suffer from this chronic disease, ill prepared for the challenges ahead. According to the New York Times, the divorce risk is higher when the wife becomes ill.[7]

It saddens me to recall numerous instances when after giving someone a PD diagnosis, the partner, sometimes of many years, would suddenly leave/abandon the patient when faced with the prospect of caring for them for a very long time. What troubled me was that this was not always in young couples; sometimes it happened in those who had been together for over twenty years, which always surprised me. These results were not unusual according to the article, which stated that when women were told they had a serious medical condition, "they became seven times more likely to become separated or divorced as men with similar health problems." I find this astounding and appalling at the same time.[8] I am sure I was not the most surprised in those relationships. I was suddenly pushed into a role not just of healthcare provider but also of a confident counselor to try to put the pieces back. Sometimes, these women and I became close friends. My job was no longer just helping them cope with a physical ailment but also how to deal with an emotional void of both receiving bad news of chronic progressive illness and of losing one's mate all at once. This was an extremely difficult task to accomplish which often required a multidisciplinary approach. From personal observation, the patients who struggled more were the ones with no support or who chose to not have ancillary therapy like counseling, etc.

How do we women with PD cope with marriage, PD, and the prospect of being divorced, separated, and widowed?

My advice comes from over sixteen years of experience as a Parkinson specialist with nearly twenty years of marriage, the last eight years spent fighting Parkinson's as an individual, and as a couple. Marriage is a very tricky and extremely fragile thing, but if you know how to care for it, it can be as solid as a rock. Not an easy task, mind you!

I want you to think of marriage and love as an empty box, or treasure chest. This is where we usually keep all our precious things from the past, and our future dreams. But, you can only draw out of this box what you have taken time to put into it. So, if you never put any love, respect, gratitude, friendship, companionship, staying power, patience, joy, laughter, communication, and openness in it, when times get hard and you go to make a withdrawal you may come up empty-handed.

No matter how long a marriage has lasted, a diagnosis of a chronic illness makes anyone feel strained and stressed, partly from concern for the loved one who is now ill, plus concern for future financial security in the midst of an illness that is unpredictable due to its progressive nature. The ability to provide for the needs of the spouse with an illness can weigh heavily. Therefore, communication is paramount concerning any area where choices can greatly impact the marriage or relationship. Remember, a marriage is made of two people so there must be accord between the two parties. If there is no communication between the partners involved, problems will not be easily solved or resolved. I have learned that both the person receiving the diagnosis and the person having the responsibility of caring for that person will immediately begin to experience the five stages of grief (the stages described in a previous chapter). You can't rush the process. Know that most likely you will not be on the same page, which can make life a little hairy! Denial, bargaining, acceptance, anger, and depression are all part of normal evolving as human beings. I put them here out of order because sometimes people may cycle in and out of any and all before reaching acceptance and learning to embrace life once again!

It is also imperative that each partner has enough time to process the information handed to them and go through the grief stages at their own pace until they reach acceptance. Everyone is different as to how long he/she takes to be able to come to terms with the gravity of the disease. For instance, I thought my husband had accepted my diagnosis of eight years. He has always been supportive and although his outlook is always positive, he shocked me recently. Not sure why, but he had spare time that particular morning so he spent a lot time reading about things that concerned my medical problems. The funny thing was that when he got up he was all upset because he FINALLY had unveiled how truly sick I really am/was! Shocker! After years of him reassuring me, I was now in a position of having to reassure him that I would be okay . . . he had concocted this whole elaborate plan for me to stay healthy, which included a whole regimen of diet, exercise, etc. I realized he never really accepted my illness, or as it happened to me last year, he probably just cycled back again in light of new medical information which he had been unaware of. He is much better now—thank goodness!

Marriages may already feel stressed from dealing with an unexpected diagnosis of chronic illness especially when this arrives at a young age and forces couples to make about-face decisions regarding their careers, family lives, etc. Marriages do better if they have endured other stressors in the past or have had a lengthy relationship prior to diagnosis as a general rule. However, unfortunately I have personally witnessed several marriages become dissolved at the sudden announcement of a spouse having a neurodegenerative disease even after twenty years of nuptials! Divorces tend to occur more frequently among young women who are newly diagnosed with PD.[9] Another study showed females to have higher rates of divorce if they were diagnosed with brain cancer, MS or PD.[10]

What this tells me is that not only are we ill equipped to face personal tragedies but as couples we are lacking the necessary coping skills and communication skills needed to overcome these life-changing events. As soon as a diagnosis is given, couples should be sent to counseling both alone and as a couple to avoid these pitfalls, something which we don't do much until it is usually too late, I am afraid.

First, we as patients must learn to look for warning signs and learn how to avoid the pitfalls that may end up taking us down the wrong road to splitsville. We must understand that we are not alone, that this is a problem of two not one, and the first place to get advice is your physician or medical team. This usually requires a multidisciplinary approach involving your doctor, a psychologist, counselor, psychiatrist, or (religious) marriage counselor. After all, we as women deal differently with stress and release different quantities of hormones than our male partners do in dealing with the same situation. We tend to want someone to fuss over us for a bit while our spouses or boyfriends may just want to move on or focus only on the material needs and ignore our emotional needs.

Furthermore, the disease itself can make us women with Parkinson's more susceptible to negative feelings especially at the onset of the disease in the early stages before medications have had a chance to start working, but also later on when medicines have been on board for a while, and certain types of medicines can cause mood swings. Therefore, these emotionally charged feelings if misdirected, not appropriately handled, or acknowledged can lead, unfortunately, to separation, which may be unwarranted if properly addressed by all parties. The spouse needs to know early on that there may be mood swings or problems with depression, which can be treated with time. Develop a plan together and set up weekly alone time to discuss stressors before they become insurmountable. Address all concerns about your relationship early on with your spouse and with your doctor and review periodically. As mentioned, if needed, seek advice from other professionals like marriage counselors, psychiatrists, psychologists, behavioral therapists, religious leaders, or support groups to avoid escalating problems. It is important to address issues both as a couple and as an individual. Short-term, intermediate, and long-term goals need to be set as a couple and as an individual to foster dreams and ambitions. You and your partner may also require treatment with antidepressants and/or anti-anxiety medications to help with coping. Also, remember to think about spiritual health for overall wellbeing as we discussed earlier, which might benefit you, your partner, and your family to help with the issue of acceptance by way of fostering love for one another. Things that may help with spiritual wellbeing are art therapy, meditation, singing in the choir, yoga, prayer, tai chi, church attendance, and enrolling in a women's prayer group or bible study. Encourage your partners to seek their own support group. It is imperative you have alone time and continue working both as individuals and as a team.

One way my husband and I have been able to cope with PD is by thinking of my illness in the following manner, especially since we are both in the medical field.

We often think of living with PD in our lives similar to the lifestyle of two medical professionals who not only share the same field but are married to one another and work in the same office! They come home day after day bringing homework problems that are the same since they share the same office and space. On top of that they share the same family issues at home—no escape! Eventually, they simply run out of new things to talk about because they are overtaken by their mutual problems, which basically converge into one big giant problem that can no longer be separated into his and hers or personal vs. work-related. This is what is meant by the old adage: "familiarity breeds contempt." It's true…you cannot expect your husband or partner to be your lover, provider, caregiver, chauffer, doctor, companion, best friend, champion, and protector 100% of the time. This is a huge burden for any one person to bear. Even the strongest among us would eventually feel the load and would want out. I feel that sometimes, we patients, especially women, may feel so insecure or devastated by the sudden change in our circumstances or life prognosis, that the grief is so profound or the depression is so big and untreated that inadvertently we drive a wedge between our spouses and us.

We need to check our emotions at least weekly and if we are finding ourselves becoming more "needy" and less independent, then I suggest we not only take action to find out what is going on by talking to our doctor, as well as make time ourselves to reenergize. My husband and I usually spin, twirl, and sometimes get dizzy and fall, yet with every change in my disease, we find a way to keep up with the rhythm of our hectic lives, some days faster than others depending on circumstances. But, no matter what, we try to keep the communication lines open and maintain sensitivity to one another's projects, ideas, and feelings, which, believe me, don't always coincide with the other's ideas, feelings, and projects!

In all marriages in general, especially those under strain due to trauma, sudden loss or chronic illness, those of us who battle PD on a daily basis need to find some alone time. We must continue to pursue our own individual interest in order to develop and grow as people. I have heard that men tend to be more loving and mindful of their wives when they have some guy time with their male friends. So by all means, don't take your husband's sense of virility and masculinity by demanding he spend all his time with you and your illness. This will only harvest resentment. Plus remember, Parkinson's is but one part of our lives, not who we are. So don't make it the center of your marriage, relationship, or life.

Having Parkinson's should not limit you from dreaming and pursuing dreams, albeit it may be different than the ones you might have planned prior to your diagnosis. Remember, we have been given a gift to be able to start anew and reinvent ourselves.

Moreover, it is imperative that each person continues to not only grow and develop as an individual with goals and dreams but also have common goals and dreams as a couple (team). These goals must be realistic and must be subject to change and modification depending on disease progression. Make those short-term, medium-term and long-term goals both as an individual and as a couple and revise them periodically to adjust for circumstances or disease changes. Flexibility on behalf of each party involved is KEY to a good marriage as well as marriage longevity when faced with adversity. Also important in maintaining love and marriage in stressful situations like dealing with Parkinson's disease is not just communication but having a sense of humor!! At times, this is more important than flexibility and as important as communication. I can honestly say that humor has kept our marriage strong through thick and thin. For as you know, humor is a great release factor and laughter inducer, which has been proven without a doubt to be the best medicine by releasing stress and building up your immune system. This is vital in preventing further decline and feeling run down.

The thing that has kept my husband and me together despite four bouts of cancer and eight years of Parkinson's is laughter and humor. He often breaks into song from a tune from *Land Before Time* when I am down and can't move and feel like a ninety-year-old—*"Even though you look like you . . . you know we like you too . . . we are family and you are one of us now!"*[11] Then my daughter typically joins in, if she is around. *"We are family and you are one of us now, we are family and you are one of us now!"* (Until we are all singing and laughing). As you might have gathered by now, we have a lot of silly songs to help us cope, which also bonds us together as a family and as a couple.

The other important source of marital discord aside from dealing with disease "24/7" or "31" as my husband calls it or "around the clock," of course, is the financial burden that comes along with caring for a chronically ill person. When someone is suddenly thrust into a life they did not expect—having to deal with the ups and downs of a person that is sick—the financial and emotional stresses can be too much to bear.

Another way I often suggest to patients and friends with PD to safeguard their marriage is to give their spouses a break, especially when caregiving or carepartnering duties become more arduous as the disease progresses in later stages. If your spouse, especially if an excellent partner and good provider, is already worried about you, your health, your emotional wellbeing, your future, your finances, your capabilities to perform activities of daily living, your health insurance, and so on ad nauseum—you do not need to worry him or her with every PD symptom you have! If you are bedbound or in end-stage PD, this is when your spouse needs some down time to be able to renew their energy to keep being able to care for you. Always surround yourself with a good circle of friends to strengthen you and lift you up.

For instance, I rely on my close friends who also have PD or friends who have family members with PD for support and companionship to events, meetings, and doctor's appointments should I need someone to drive me or be a chaperone, if I can't travel alone due to medical reasons. In this fashion, my husband's job is not disrupted nor does he have to be with me "31" and we can continue being independent of one another with our own duties and responsibilities. However, of course there are times when he MUST step in because I am unable to fulfill certain roles at home as a wife or mother due to my illness and no one else is available to help. We prefer to keep these kinds of disruptions to a minimum whenever possible so that this is the exception rather than the rule in order to try to maintain normalcy in our daughter's life as much as possible, which is particularly important during her formative years.

Although my husband supports me and stands by my side 100% with all my activities and projects, he does not very often participate in my Parkinson's events. That's our compromise and one of his coping mechanisms. I, on the other hand, view it as continuation of my profession. I attend my PD conferences on my own as I did when I was working just as he attends his when necessary to keep up his license requirements. Although I am more dependent on him than I have been in the past, we try to maintain our own individual dreams, passions, and goals just as we always have, but with the understanding that due to my illness, which tends to have its ups and downs, we have to be more flexible than before. This requires some juggling of life's demands at a moment's notice. This is not always easy since there is always one person that is able to cope faster or bounce quicker than another. This is usually me, so I don't push too much after an unexpected downfall to allow him to come to terms with it, which usually takes the form of overprotectiveness until I can prove that I will be fine on my own again! This, however, does not diminish his worrying, which I deeply appreciate.

So, you must be in tune with your partner's emotions and reactions and understand his/her reasoning for doing things to avoid hurt feelings and misunderstandings.

The important thing to remember from all this is that in marriage, as in life, you have to fight for what you want and love. Nothing worthwhile ever lasts if you are not willing to put in the time and deposit into that empty box what you may need to withdraw at a future time. If you have a spouse who is accepting of your illness and is willing to stay by your side, be grateful, for this is half the battle.

- Learn to embrace life and your marriage DESPITE PD.
- Learn to make a difference in someone's life, even if it's just your own.

My husband still has times when he wants to wring my neck, because as he puts it, I like to play "lawyer ball" with him, pulling a "Clinton," since sometimes I don't truly remember things due to my medications. When asked about a particular situation that I don't have all the facts clear in my mind, I often reply: "I may or may not have done such and such a thing. I do not have a clear recollection of the events; therefore, I can't answer!" This is the God's honest truth! This drives him nuts, understandably, but I honestly can't help him during such instances. On the other hand, I get frustrated at him if a new event in my disease occurs which I have not fully processed or may be experiencing denial or anger with, while he has already moved on with our life and is in full acceptance mode. With every new incident or decline in my disease (and in every patient's illness) there is always a readjustment or grieving process that has to take place, which everyone forgets about! Therefore, allow yourself and your partner time to grieve, and talk openly and frequently!

Remember, even the strongest person needs encouragement, support, and loving embraces or they, too, will crumble eventually!

The topic at home should not be all about Parkinson's, doctors, or bills. PD is but a small, albeit significant, part of our lives but is NOT the only thing directing it or stressing it and IT should NOT be. Allowed center stage, there are kids to raise, family to tend to, careers to grow, goals to pursue, futures to plan, and memories to make as a family and as a couple. Build on one another's strengths in order to keep moving forward to prevent being stuck, or worse, fall apart!

But sometimes despite all the churning, you only end up exhausted and empty-handed without an ounce of cream in hand to show for all your hard work. What then? You have done all the things I talked about, but your partner is still not willing to make an effort to meet you halfway; he is not interested in moving forward, refuses therapy, and shows no interest in having a life together. Then it is time to move on for the sake of your physical, mental, and spiritual wellbeing! He simply may not possess the right coping skills, and lack of interest in acquiring these skills is what makes marriage a failure. What makes it more painful is that we do not live in a vacuum where the only issue we have to confront and deal with is Parkinson's

Regardless of years of marriage, to suddenly realize that the single most important person whom you love was supposed to stand by your side for better or for worse chose to leave when you needed them the most can be emotionally and physically paralyzing and numbing! But I am here to tell you that you are not alone and you are better off, particularly if that partner is no longer vested in your happiness and wellbeing!

Good news: there is someone else great out there for you and even better to know that the second marriages of chronically ill patients are more stable and successful because the people involved are fully aware of each other's limitations, condition, disabilities, etc. and already anticipate a financial and emotional toll on their life; thus they are fully invested in the relationship from the start.[12] So, if you are not in a relationship and want one, go for it! You are beautiful!!! Moreover, as modern women we have access to education, training, and employment, which our mothers and grandmothers were not privy to; therefore, we are able to live creative, independent lives if we want to.

9

Sex and Parkinson's: The Bedroom Goddess

"Sex is emotion in motion"
~ Mae West

This chapter more than any other is about making the impossible possible! As all of you know, sexuality is an intrinsic part of who we are as human beings; it's what differentiates us from the other mammalian species. As Henry Louis Mencken once quipped, *"Life without sex might be safer but it would be unbearably dull. It is the sex instinct which makes women seem beautiful...and men seem wise and brave...Throttle it, denaturalize it, take it away, and human existence would be reduced to the prosaic, laborious, boresome, imbecile level of life in an anthill."*[1] Strong powerful words. If we are to believe in this statement, no wonder we as humans spend so much time worrying, thinking, and pursuing sexual pleasure! Therefore, when our sexuality is threatened or altered, especially in the context of a stable monogamous relationship, it can wreak havoc in our lives. Lack thereof may very well threaten our very own existence and happiness. This is true for both men and women alike. However, I personally believe that we as women tend to overlook problems in this area more often than our partners do. Yet, there is no denying that sex and sexual intimacy play a crucial role in all of our lives.

Sexual issues can be a huge problem in any marriage or partnership, but even more critical in people living with PD when nearly 87% of people with this disorder professed to having some type of sexual problem according to a survey of 351 PD patients.[2] Furthermore, because of its personal nature it is something that has to be dealt with, not just in a timely matter but also very delicately, to avoid issues of guilt, self-doubt, blame, loss of self-esteem, or even self-deprecation in either partner.

To complicate matters a bit further, we know, or at least have a notion deep down in our souls that men prefer a woman who is not afraid to try new things in the bedroom. The problem may come head-on when the woman we once were: adventurous, feisty, thrill-seeker, may begin to morph into the so-called PD "personality type": rigid, socially awkward, depressive, overly controlling, morally rigid, and stoic because of lack of dopamine or other medications, no longer finding pleasure in the old things.[3]

Therefore, all people with Parkinson's have to cope with a contorted labyrinth regarding intimacy, sex, and sensuality.

It is not uncommon for us women to experience fluctuations in our libidos due to hormone changes brought about by medications, illnesses, contraceptives, menstrual cycle, menopause, or childbirth. Those of us with PD may also experience decrease in lubrication, causing painful intercourse, 18% of the PD cases, and may even have trouble achieving orgasms.[4, 5] Women with PD make up the minority of those with increased sexual urges, only 8% of the cases, as opposed to the great majority of men with PD who described feeling very hypersexual most of the time.[6] Over the course of your illness, however, sexual feelings or desire may heighten by falling dopamine levels or may be induced by some dopamine agonists.[7] Moreover, changes in our physical and emotional life due to Parkinson's can lead to us to have a less than ideal sex life.

Now, recall that we women with Parkinson's manifest symptoms differently but also deal with them in different ways and progress in a very unique manner particular to our own gender. For instance, we Parkinson's women, although with less overall motor deficits as per UPDRS, we seem to have a lot more disability and difficulty in achieving the appropriate quality of life to keep us happy or to be able to maintain the status quo. This is partly due to increased tendency to develop non-motor symptoms like depression, which tends to color our overall view of the world. The depression can cause us to feel less attractive, have decreased desire, and more difficulty achieving orgasm. Much of a woman's pleasure is, after all, in the brain, all wrapped up in emotions.[8] Hence, if your head tells you that you are unattractive because you are shaky, stiff, or dyskinetic, you are not going to feel much like enjoying sex no matter how much you love your partner. If your brain and mind are not feeling it, it is not happening no matter how hot he may be.

After initial diagnosis, it is important to allow yourself a period of adjustment in your intimacy life as a couple, as both of you learn to deal and cope with the ramifications of dealing with a long-term illness, particularly one that is progressive in nature. As the disease progresses and new challenges arise, be open to the need for readjustment or reevaluation in the manner in which your sex life is conducted. Sexual intimacy does not have to stop but may require new understanding of what is pleasurable and what is not. Also given the progressive changes in dexterity and flexibility, new techniques may have to be instituted. Be open to new ideas and new positions.

Maintain lines of communication open at all times between you and your mate as well as between yourself and your physician, so he or she can provide counseling along with needed medications to help cope with any troubling situations which may ensue along the way.

Unfortunately, despite all the sex talk that we seem to be surrounded by in the media daily, which includes overt propaganda and sexual innuendos, there still appears to be a taboo of speaking about one's own sexual issues or dilemmas to one's own friends, much less to one's own doctor(s). This is unless he/she initiates conversation and even then, it is usually a very awkward one-sided discussion. We are reluctant to discuss our personal and private affairs with very few people, if any, but rarely are comfortable discussing problems or concerns with our own healthcare providers even if we know them well and trust them, for fear of being labeled or judged. We must get over this self-deprecating image of inferiority when it comes to issues of sexual dysfunction or intimacy and accept that it is just as real and normal a part of our lives as having tremors or slowness when we have Parkinson's disease. If we want to feel better about ourselves and once again find joy and pleasure in our relationships with our partners, we must be able to discuss the issues in an open, no-judgmental way to receive the right treatment or counseling.

In my years of practice, I discovered a great deal of hesitation in bringing up the subject, particularly in the older PD populations, independent of gender, even though this was the foremost important issue in their lives and reason for seeking medical advice. Among three thousand five men and women interviewed in the US about the frequency of sexual activity, it revealed the crucial role sexual intimacy plays in all of our lives, independent of age; it was just as important for middle-aged couples as it was to elderly couples. In individuals between the ages of fifty-seven to sixty-four, 73% were sexually active; 53% in those age sixty-five to seventy-four; and 26% were still enjoying a full sex life of those were over seventy-five.[9]

Sex among elders around the world was just as important. In a study of Swedish men, 98% said "sex is important."[10] In my practice, the subject was often skirted around or brought out at the last minute as we had already closed our conversation and were walking out the door! In my practice, it was the men who not only typically discussed the topic but also asked for treatment, usually insisting on getting "Viagra" or the "blue pill" over any other brand. Some even claimed that this was the ONLY medication they needed for their Parkinson's disease, revealing the importance of sexual intimacy and perhaps unveiling something much more interesting about why we are so addicted to sexual activity as human beings, especially for PD patients. It turns out that when we achieve orgasm during sexual intercourse, a large quantity of dopamine is released from our brains—the one essential chemical we Parkinson's individuals lack! So, you can say that sex is not only healthy but necessary to maintain wellbeing in a non-pharmaceutical way.[11]

It is also very important to recall that both women and men with PD suffer from sexual dysfunction as a result of both the non-motor effects of Parkinson's disease but also as a result of medication side effects. Since we have very different coping skills than our male PD friends, it is these coping skills that set us apart from one another, at times making us act completely irrational. In general, men gamble and women overeat or shop.

Sexual behaviors and gambling have been related to intake of dopamine agonists. However, these appear to be much more common in men than in women.[12] So, as you can see, women's PD can have a more profound impact on sexuality on an emotional level, as opposed to men's PD, which tends to have more of an overt problem; nevertheless, either one can lead to strain on any relationship. However, unlike most men with PD, the sexual behaviors of sexuality and intimacy in women with PD, in my experience, appear to be intricately tied to self-worth. This inner turmoil can then fuel the depression.

I know we have a long way to go in the medical field in dealing with these problems; in particular in the context of Parkinson's disease, because until recently we did not even know these problems existed.

Despite the fact that most of us know and hear about sexual problems being an issue in Parkinson's disease, the majority of patients in a study done, looking at 351 individuals who openly admitted having sexual problems, 49% never even discussed the issues with their physicians. [13]

Personally, I had a real revelation in this department, both as a patient and as a former Parkinson's specialist, realizing the enormity and complexity of the issue surrounding PD and sexuality. Recently, I discovered that the medications I was prescribed were making me depressed. Subsequently, I was experiencing decreased libido and sexual drive. I found myself initially being embarrassed and reluctant to discuss the subject with my neurologist, who is not only my colleague but also an old friend. This hesitancy on my part really got me thinking about this irony, given that I as a physician have broached this subject with my patients many times during the course of my career. Why was I having such a hard time? It came down to the fact of my own insecurities. It seems it is a lot easier to discuss a single problem in the context of a "normal' life but when you perceive your world is changing and falling apart, as is the case with Parkinson's disease, talking about a symptom that is as personal as nothing else in this world, it can make you feel extremely vulnerable and exposed even more so than you already do because of loss of independence, previous abilities, etc. As I discovered, having these conversations are a matter of self-love and self-worth; if you value your happiness, you will be open to discuss ways of becoming whole again.

You can't get help if you don't let others know about the problem. Physicians won't understand the magnitude of the problem until we start sharing our problems with them.

In my instance, the decreased libido led to a state of depression, creating a catch-22 scenario. The more depressed I got the less interested I became in sexual intimacy, but that did not exclude the need for other non-sexual contact. My husband on the other hand saw my lack of sexual interest as lack of desire for other areas in our life, such as couple time for emotional bonding. The result was that for the first time in my adult life, I began to get very clingy, needy, and overtly suspicious of my husband as well as extremely jealous. It was driving me crazy to feel this way since I had always been an independent woman and very trusting of my husband. My state of mind was akin to that of a child who has been "sugared up," or has a paradoxical or opposite reaction to a medication, like Benadryl. They are supposed to get sleepy and sedated but instead they end up irritable, inconsolable, and unable to rest or stop the tears because they have no emotional control over their bodies, their environment, or their situation. Such was my emotional state at the time. I felt like a ship in the middle of the ocean, thrust about by the high winds without any control whatsoever, at the mercy of outside forces. Believe me, this is not a good feeling! Like that inconsolable child who desperately needs someone to hold him or to rescue him from a sinking ship, when someone does offer to help, the person drowning will resist to the bitter end until they succumb to exhaustion. This is precisely how I felt—completely "out of control," knowing full well this was not normal, NOT me; yet I could not stop acting or feeling overwhelmed and out of sorts. Even worse, I was beginning to foster feelings of resentment towards my husband. I felt he had somehow betrayed me for not doing more, or understanding why I was acting this way. This is an extremely dangerous place to be when we begin to assign blame to others for our unhappiness, expecting others to solve our emotional crises. If spouses do not understand or know the person well, this typically leads to separation or divorce. I was experiencing completely irrational behavior and was out of character. Although I hated the feelings, I could not help but feel the wave of decreased confidence, self-esteem and vitality. I was on the verge of a nervous breakdown. At some point, I found myself staring into a deep abyss of loneliness and hopelessness that I had never encountered before in my entire life. Thank God for faith, my husband, laughter, and strong communication between us, as well as for my husband's patience and insight. Even though I felt he was not understanding or noticing me and my problems, he truly was in tune with my mood changes. He was the first to recognize that this behavior was out of character for me. And as any good husband does, he quickly went in search of a solution to my problem to get me back to myself. If it had not been for my faith and my husband's love, I could not have weathered the storm.

At that time, our marriage hit a big bump in the road. Had it not been for a big dose of humor and laughter injected into our chaotic lives, it could have had a potentially disastrous outcome.

Communication is the key, along with a big heap of love and compassion, to overcoming any situation of whatever magnitude.

Afterwards, my husband illustrated my behavior by recalling a story of a friend who, in a state of severe depression that she, too, became extremely jealous and possessive of her husband to the point that one day she was so determined to go and find her husband. She was convinced he was having an affair, so she drove off in search of him to prove to herself that this was the case. When she arrived she did not find his truck, so she began circling about, becoming more and more enraged with every turn, only to realize after what seemed an eternity that she was driving HIS TRUCK! After my husband reminded me of this story, he said, "I can totally see you doing this," at which point I had to laugh. I was so upset with him and my mind was so clouded at the time, I could totally see myself doing the same thing and feeling completely foolish.

It turned out that the combination of medications had brought about this sudden and drastic personality change. Once we changed medications there were no more feelings of hopelessness, low self-esteem or complete obsession with my husband's whereabouts. He was most relieved since I stopped calling his office so much during the day and he could actually work in peace again! Most importantly, I was no longer a basket case, crying at a drop of a hat (akin to the Mexican mythological creature, La Llorona, crying in every corner). I was lucky to have a husband that cared enough. Someone else might have just thought I was crazy, not cared, or worse, filed for divorce.

The lesson here is fourfold:

1. I can't stress enough about the importance of laughter in a relationship; after all, it is the best medicine for the soul and helps to reduce stress, build up the immune system, along with adding longevity to your years.
2. An open communication between all parties involved is of the utmost importance.
3. If things suddenly change in any area of your life, like sexual function, mental instability, depression or cognitive changes, seek immediate medical help.
4. Love, respect, and mutual understanding are the keys to weathering any storm within a marriage.

Money and sexual intimacy problems are big factors in ending relationships. Perhaps, if we could find a way to continue or improve sexual intimacy, divorce rates among the chronically ill would not be as high. After all, a study revealed that the benefits of maintaining or having an intimate and sexual relationship extended well beyond the bedroom into other spheres of life. Some of the benefits reported as a result of having an intimate and sexual relationship with your partner are emotional and physical relaxation, increased confidence, as well as self-esteem, along with an increase in vitality. Plus, since many of us with Parkinson's have pain of some type, there is also an added bonus of experiencing pain relief.[13]

Finally, only through intimacy will you be able to achieve greater life satisfaction and quality of life. For many of us women who operate more in the FEELING realm, having more intimacy could help diminish some of the negative symptoms that come about with PD, like anxiety.[14, 15] When we are happy, we tend to feel more fulfilled, appreciated, less disabled, less like a victim and more like a victor, which in turn leads to an increase in expression of gratitude towards our partners.[16, 17] This latter aspect is crucial in maintaining the glue and keeping that treasure chest or keepsake box filled for future withdrawals. When gratitude is freely displayed, caregiving becomes less of a burden and more of an act of love.

It is just as important for us women with PD as for men with Parkinson's to focus and spend time on four domains: [18]

1. Intimate time with our partners. This includes both physical and emotional bonding and sharing.
2. Couple time away from family, kids, work, etc. dedicated to improve and foster togetherness and oneness. This is the number one area that must be fostered, particularly in couples with chronic illnesses, paying close attention to the needs of your partner—building trust, and depositing respect, love, devotion, and thoughtfulness into that empty box to be drawn on at times of duress, and to allow couples to weather even the strongest of storms.
3. Sexual time.
4. Personal time to develop. We all need alone time to grow as individuals, to nurture our minds and souls, and to gather strength to be able to cope with life stressors. We need our own dreams.

All domains are equally important and should be fostered equally to be a well-balanced individual.

Another factor that makes dealing with sexual issues in Parkinson's complicated is the notion that some people believe that experiencing sexual dysfunction is the most disabling and demoralizing feature of living with PD, especially within the context of marriage.[19] Our thoughts control our actions; if we go around thinking we are defeated, then we have already lost the battle . . . we *will* be defeated. But if you think you can overcome this pesky and inconvenient problem and make it a challenge to conquer, then you will be victorious.

I admit sometimes we may feel schizophrenic when it comes to sexual desires and wants in relation to PD; on one hand we can have wild, erotic dreams brought on by the effects of medications, especially the dopamine agonists. Personally, I find that these medications increase libido when we allow them to "wear off", acting more like a withdrawal effect, plus they seem to enhance the person's natural state or inner feelings or desires at that time. For instance, if you and your lover have not had sexual intercourse or sexual encounters for a period of time, what I have encountered is a heightening of desire induced by medication. But if you are regularly sexually active, the medications have little effect on this system. Then you may experience decreased lubrication due to Parkinson's and PD medications, leading to painful intercourse and making you confused as to whether or not you should venture down this road.

Okay, so you now find yourself in a heightened state and you and your partner are willing to make a go of it, but there is still the actual physical act to carry out. You realize this may take some doing due to clumsiness in fine motor control during lovemaking or increased tremors with enhanced arousal during sexual intercourse. Creativity is extremely important during this stage.

As one courageous woman with YOPD found out firsthand, having Parkinson's and intimacy simultaneously could be a tricky thing to handle: "Prior to diagnosis, whenever I would climax, my right arm would flop around like a chicken with its head cut off. I could not control it. After I was on meds, things were back to normal." Yet, she and her husband found a way to make things work.

Nevertheless, because you know that sex is important to maintain unity of a marriage and know men like to have some variety and be surprised, you are determined to make the impossible possibly happen. So you decide you will spark things up a bit in your marriage. One particular morning for instance, you are feeling absolutely *diva-licious* and want to give your spouse a proper sendoff to work. Therefore, you conspire to get up extra early since not only is he an early bird but he also leaves quite early. But this means your medicines have not had time to kick in yet! Your spouse is obviously excited and aroused by show of interest and enthusiasm but then it becomes a comedy of errors since you are completely stiff and can't bend your neck or torso. You are even unable to sit down without falling over, much less go down on the floor due to your own torso's rigidity. Finally, with much effort and willpower, you muster enough energy to bend just right to take his manhood in your mouth, only to discover that the medications still have not kicked in enough to get rid of the severe bruxism and oral dystonia that is plaguing you. Thus, inadvertently in the midst of passion your mouth locks involuntarily, accidentally biting down harder than intended; thus, causing pain instead of pleasure. Fortunately, you thank your lucky stars that you were able to unclench your jaw; otherwise, the very idea of having to call the paramedics is humiliating enough, much less having to make a trip down to the emergency room where you know for sure you will NEVER be forgotten! So, what started as an arousing, stimulating event between two loving, consenting adults becomes a less-than-desirable event and more humorous than erotic with a great sigh of relief because of potential outcome. Now, for years to come, you will recall this memorable experience and might even start to laugh, deepening the bond between two people that love one another.

Sometimes what starts as a playful, loving act suddenly becomes a challenge, like climbing a mountain; something you must achieve to prove you ARE capable? But, with each passing moment you wonder if it is worth it.

Women might feel depressed, frustrated, and insecure, especially if there is no communication or empathy from their spouse. Without the support, these feelings can quickly escalate to loneliness and feelings of sexual dissatisfaction and self-deprecation.

We must learn to not only be aware of the problem but also understand the reasons we experience these behaviors and be able to find clear solutions to keep our world from becoming dull, unbearable, chaotic, and out of control. We have to learn to speak our minds and not be afraid of being judged by others or appearing weak or vulnerable, or less in control. In fact, when we take charge of our situations and understand the root of the problems, we become empowered and are able to rise above our circumstances. Learn to use your symptoms to your advantage, like using your rest tremors to pleasure your partner. Don't be afraid to experiment and try new things to make it easier for your condition and to keep the mystery and flame alive. If you need some inspiration, I suggest renting the movie *Love & Other Drugs*, released in 2010. It is loosely based on a true story about a Pfizer sales representative who meets a young women with early onset PD who is having some of these issues so she handles her insecurities overtly sexual. Very steamy scenes for you and your partner to enjoy but more importantly it has a bigger message of "sticking-to-it-ive-ness" and learning to cope with a disabling illness. When this movie came out, I realized that the Parkinson's community missed a big opportunity to raise awareness about a still largely misdiagnosed disease, especially in young people and women, but also to talk about salient issues afflicting people of all ages with PD. However, the movie took a more personal stage after I did my first Unity Walk in New York in Central Park, as a People with Parkinson's Advisory Committee (PPAC) member for the Parkinson's Disease Foundation. One of the people I got to meet that year, aside from Michael J. Fox, was none other than the young lady, Maggie Murdock, on whom the story was based. She told me about her struggles with PD at such a young age and having such severe rest tremors. I often think of her. Happy to have met her and saddened, too, because she was still so very shaky she could barely stand, talk, or use her hands in this era of DBS treatments and other great medical advances. She also handed me a poem she had written about her condition, which I put for safekeeping and apparently stored so well that I have not been able to retrieve it due to old age or PD. So, watching this movie might help you gain some further insight into PD, marriage, relationships, and sex. I also feel that the movie captures the true essence of PD support groups.

Finally, like Maggie, don't be afraid to speak your mind. Talk about your needs, desires, and expectations with your partner and do what makes you happy. Communication is not just a two-way street but it is also an intricate love dance of two. You cannot tango with only one person. No wonder the Tango is considered the "dance of love." Partners move rhythmically in unison with barely a ray of light passing through them. Initially, until both partners learn to trust the other, there is a lot of stepping on toes, back pulling, and having the wind knocked out of us at the slightest movement.[20] I guess it is no coincidence that the "Tango" is the dance that has proved to be the most beneficial for those of us who have Parkinson's. This is because you have to go by instinct and learn to trust someone else to lead rather than your own brain bypassing those faulty connections in the basal ganglia, until you are able to move normally through someone else's control.[21, 22] Next time you feel that you cannot possibly enjoy some one-on-one time with your mate because you are a little off and a little tired, remember that there is always room for experimentation! You may be surprised as to what you can do with a little imagination. Channel your inner diva and shine on with a touch of edible "Dust-up Kissable Body Shimmer" from Victoria's Secret. It comes in marshmallow, candy, and cocoa flavors, the latter being the stuff that the gods from ancient times dreamed of, and may help ignite that inner sparkle.[23]

10

Parkinson Medication Effect on the Female Patient

"The only real mistakes are the ones we don't learn from."
~ Author Unknown

From both a physician and patient standpoint, I have noticed that aside from typical side effects related to dopamine and dopamine agonists such as dizziness, nausea, and blood pressure alterations, sometimes the medications can affect the female constitution in unique ways because the sex of a person taking the medications does matter! Sometimes you just don't know if you are coming or going; you feel like you are losing your mind. You have gotten on a roller coaster to which there seems to be no end in sight. As a woman, particularly as we get closer to menopause, we start to wonder if all our symptoms are hormonal or worst yet, sometimes our doctors ASSUME all of our symptoms are hormonal, which can be a very dangerous assumption. As we have been discussing all along, our hormones DO play a role in our disease! Furthermore, some of the symptoms caused by decreased hormones, like fatigue, anxiety, difficulty sleeping, weight changes (especially gain), can all be seen as a result of Parkinson's and a potential side effect of the medications. Plus, remember that we women tend to have more side effects with medications overall.[1] This scenario only worsens as we age. This is when it is particularly important to have open communication with your physician and alert him/her to any sudden changes, since no one knows your body better than you do. Keep a diary; this will help better determine the cause.

We all know too well that Parkinson's medications have their own unique set of side effects that can alter a patient's mood and constitution, disrupt sleep patterns, and even alter a patient's unique chemical balance, which makes each and every one of us who we are: an artist, a doctor, a thrill seeker, or an introvert. This is all determined by the amount of neurotransmitters (dopamine, serotonin etc.) you have in your brain. We have heard that some people are more likely to commit crimes because in utero they have more exposure to serotonin and thus become desensitized in the frontal lobes.[2] Hence, when we introduce drugs to treat neurological diseases that affect the mind, we are changing the natural order of things. Therefore, we need to be prepared to recognize what's acceptable, what's not, and when something can be potentially harmful.

Recent studies have suggested that dopamine disorders like Parkinson's can interfere with the natural oxytocin levels of the brain, leading to sexual behavioral problems, addiction, and depression.[3] While oxytocin controls the effects of dopamine, dopamine also exerts control back on oxytocin so when there is less oxytocin we may feel more out of control, worsening the "negative" symptoms associated with PD.[4]

Interestingly, sexual and addictive behaviors occur more often in men while depressive symptoms are more common in women[5]. This perhaps points to the fact that dopamine is crucial in maintaining the hormonal equilibrium and when dopamine no longer is available, even the loss of that small amount of oxytocin in male brains can wreak havoc.

Orgasmic Dysfunction in Women with PD

As we discussed previously, sexual behaviors affect both men and women. Parkinson's itself can cause these problems, but some medications have been attributed to causing sexual problems, some more than others. For instance, rasagiline (Azilect) seems to increase and heighten sexual dreams in some women, especially at the start of the medication. Along with this heightened sexual desire comes increased libido. This side effect in my experience usually tapers off rather quickly within a week of taking the medication. However, in my experience, if patients continue to experience a heightened libido in a scenario of an "off" state or withdrawal effect, such as occurring at the end of a dose, it usually implies that they are mirroring the patient's inner feelings and desires, i.e., if someone is in need of sexual intimacy, then they will have heightened libido. Azilect has also been reported to cause women to experience spontaneous orgasms.[6] You may think this is a good thing, but this type of occurrence is known as "orgasmic dysfunction."[7] Spontaneous orgasm is the "condition of experiencing an orgasm in the absence of any sexual stimulation."[8] These episodes, however, may be so frequent that it could potentially be very painful. I am a testament to this; just recently, I began to have break-through pain and increasing my Neupro and Stalevo did little for the pain. Azilect has always worked well, but I noticed that it no longer was lasting as long as it had at the beginning. So, I was discussing this issue with one of my colleagues, and he told me that in his practice he was using up to 2 mg of this medication, which had been a studied dose, with excellent results. Subsequently I upped my dose to 1.5 mg a day, which immediately got rid of my pain, and I could function normally again. I was ecstatic, until two weeks later when I began having excruciating pain in my nether regions. Day and night I was experiencing these bursts of activity unlike before. Previously, they had been pleasant and spontaneous, now they were lasting a long time and getting more painful each time. Remembering what I had written before and previously experienced, I opted to suspend medicine for a couple of days and then taper down to my previous lower dose. Symptoms have not returned!

Unfortunately, because this area lacks understanding and is unexplored, we don't yet have all the answers; but given my experience and that of at least another woman I know, this phenomenon could be considered an idiosyncratic reaction at best or common side effect of Azilect in women at worst, especially in those of us who have other underlying illnesses such as diabetes, thyroid disease, and neurological diseases, or autonomic dysfunction involving the pelvic floor nerves because according to literature these are the diseases that predispose women to having spontaneous painful orgasms.[8] Until recently, this phenomenon was unperceived or unrelated to Parkinson's or Parkinson's medications. To date, there has been a single report of Azilect triggering this sexual dysfunction.[9] A women with YOPD described having spontaneous orgasms, as many as five to twenty episodes a day. She also experienced a state of "hyperarousal."[10]

We know that similar effects can occur with other drugs that bind the dopamine receptor, such as cocaine, so we should not be entirely surprised that these medications, which modulate and bind to dopamine receptors even more directly, can have similar effects on individuals.[11] However, because there are so many factors that could pre-dispose one to experience this orgasmic dysfunction, we cannot be entirely certain that Azilect alone is the culprit or if it works synergistically in the presence of other diseases. Only time will tell. But, should you experience these bizarre phenomena while on any PD medication, particularly if painful, make sure to report the events to the drug company as well as your physician. In this fashion, the pharmaceutical company can begin a registry documenting these side effects.

PMS/Menstrual Cycle in Women with PD

On a different subject not entirely unrelated, dopamine can interfere with hormones such as oxytocin. Therefore, it is not entirely surprising that the menstrual cycle of a woman with Parkinson's can potentially be affected as do other symptoms accompanying the disease during a woman's cycle. I along with many women whom I have treated and interacted with have confirmed this to be true. They have stated repeatedly that the Parkinson's symptoms, both motor and non-motor, seem to worsen during their menstrual cycle. In fact, according to the European Parkinson's Disease Association (EPDA), eleven out of twelve women experience worsening of Parkinson's symptoms and reduced effectiveness of their medication during the premenstrual syndrome (PMS) and menstrual cycle. The symptoms that appear to worsen are tremors, rigidity, and dyskinesia.[12] The recommendation in this case is treatment of PMS first. But, your doctor may also need to increase the doses of dopamine during these particular periods of time. As a personal observation in myself, my grandmother, and in my own patients, I found that increasing medications temporarily during the body's or individual's stressful time, whether internal or external, helps maintain equilibrium and prevent disease progression in the short-term as well as maintain quality of life with symptom control even during stressful situations. In other words, by increasing medications as needed for a brief period of time, you are avoiding and preventing fluctuations due to stress on the body.

If your menstrual cycle worsens with PD, talk to your doctor about contraceptives such as Mirena IUDs, progesterone-only pills that allow you to breast feed; changing medications; hysterectomy without removal of the ovaries, etc. But, for the increased affective disorder that sometimes accompanies a women's menstrual cycle, such as increased sadness, depression, tearfulness, moodiness, and fatigue, which could be compounded by Parkinson's disease especially if other symptoms are also worsening during the cycle, you may also want to consider an antidepressant like an SSRI (Selective Serotonin Reuptake Inhibitor) to be taken only during the PMS period just like dopamine, three days before and two days into the cycle.

Furthermore, it appears that women with PD suffer worsening menstrual symptoms after their PD diagnosis. This was the case for me, but I never did relate at the time. Common menstrual symptoms that appear to be worse are those related to pain and increased bleeding. [13] Women with Parkinson's tend to have an increase in body dysmorphic syndrome after diagnosis. Thus, they are left feeling a lot less attractive, which may be the cause for the disparity seen between men and women's PD "negative" symptoms of unfulfillment, anxiety, and depression. If we understand that this could be related at least in part to hormone effect in our bodies and treat it accordingly, then perhaps we might not see ourselves as woman altering our personal fashion and style to accommodate or cover up these feelings of inferiority or inadequacy.

Instead, we could see all PD women embracing their inner beauty and their individual femininity.

This is why it is extremely important to follow my tips on living and embracing PD as a DIVA to avoid falling into a trap of feeling less than the beautiful woman that you are—Parkinson's and ALL!! Don't forget to maintain some mystery in your marriage even if you are having all these issues. Do not feel you have to tell your partner EVERYTHING! They will thank you!

What is more difficult to grasp for those that are not in the same playing field as women who suffer with PD is the life disruption caused by having irregular menses or painful menses. Imagine being stiff, shaky, or dyskinetic now because of Parkinson's and some of the Parkinson's medications, but you are also doomed to have excessive bleeding, forcing you to go to the bathroom to change your undergarments at least ten times a day. This is assuming that your bladder is cooperating; otherwise, you may double or triple the number of visits to the bathroom. At this point, having a period can be an insurmountable task. One also assumes that the person dealing with these issues has enough dexterity to be able to accomplish such tasks of changing frequently without getting tangled or staining one's undergarments, leading many women with PD like myself to consider surgical intervention, i.e., hysterectomy, or other medical options to stop the insanity that comes with irregular menstrual cycles, especially when Parkinson's symptoms worsen every single month and periods become irregular, which only leads to more fatigue due to secondary anemia.

Migraines and PD

Now add to this the fact that menstruating women are more likely to have illnesses like migraines. Plus, some of you women may already experience "catamenial migraines", headaches associated with menstruation, a few days before and during menstrual cycle. After all, migraine incidence is more common than diabetes and asthma put together in this country.[14] Therefore, medications that can trigger headaches and migraines, such as Stalevo and L-dopa can greatly influence the types of reactions we have to medicines compared to our male Parkinson's friends of the same age. After all, you already may be experiencing worsening PMS-related PD symptoms; do you really need a headache as well to render you incapacitated? Take it from someone who has had migraines all her life. Migraines can incapacitate you for hours and days, if they are severe. Do we really need this when we also have PD to deal with? No of course not!

We must be aware that certain medications can exacerbate migraines. But if you are prone to migraines already, some of the Parkinson's symptoms such as having a stiff neck or neck dystonia may also exacerbate migraines. It is important to recognize these triggers because they will add to a young woman with Parkinson's disability and general malaise. Therefore, I recommend that if you suffer from a headache thirty minutes to an hour after taking medications, especially with nausea, light, and noise sensitivity, first make sure it is not due to a sudden elevated blood pressure. Then treat it as a migraine if there is a history of migraines. It is best to maintain a headache diary. I recommend, however, that you discuss with your physician any and all new symptoms after starting a medication before altering your medication regimen. In my experience, Levodopa, particularly in the form of Stalevo, has been more likely to cause or exacerbate migraines than the dopamine agonists or as Sinemet.

Interestingly, new data has recently surfaced which suggests that migraines, especially those with auras, could double the risk for developing PD.[15] Furthermore, this study, which followed six thousand individuals ages thirty-three to sixty-five for a period of twenty-five years, revealed that women with migraines with aura were more likely to have a family history of PD, compared to those without history of headaches.[16] This is fascinating since both my grandmother and I had migraines with aura and subsequently developed PD! I wonder if it skips a generation. It must, since my mother is asymptomatic. The rate of penetrance would be of particular value and importance to researchers as well as be able to predict who is at risk. Since penetrance measures the portion of individuals who carry a particular variant like the LLRK2 gene that then results in an associated trait like Parkinson's, or Parkinson's and migraines.[17] Sometimes in nature, the same identical genes will result in different outcomes or trait—be LLRK2 and not develop PD for instance. This is the tough part for scientists to decipher. So, only time will tell if my daughter, who has classic migraines, is at higher risk of getting Parkinson's because of family history and will develop the disease as well. I pray to God not! The next question, of course, is can we do anything to stop or prevent this outcome? All these questions still need to be addressed by researchers in the field.

Furthermore, if migraines are a risk for developing Parkinson's down the road, do we expect to see more women developing Parkinson's? Vice versa—do we also expect those women who already have the disease and a history of migraine to be more susceptible to an increase in breakthrough headaches with medications used to treat Parkinson's? This is purely based on the fact that migraines affect more women than men out of the 12% of US population believed to be suffering from migraines.[18] This is another reason why we women with PD that may have migraines or history of migraines need to keep a more accurate account of our own headaches and sharing this information with our physicians.

Vaginal Infections/Inflammation in Women with PD

Although not frequently reported, just like orgasms (once again this is from personal experience) Azilect appears to be in the lead as the culprit for recurrent vaginitis (inflammation of the vagina causing discharge, itching and pain), vaginosis (bacterial infection commonly with gardnerella, and yeast, which can cause the same symptoms but not the unique "fish odor" discharge seen with gardnerella. Because gardnerella vaginitis can be an STD (sexually transmitted disease), it could potentially wreak havoc in your relationship with your partner if you suddenly have this and think your partner has been stepping out on you. This is where trust in a partner and communication are extremely important! This has been reported as an adverse effect with the intake of Azilect.[19] Although risk factors for vaginitis are multiple sex partners, cigarette smoking, intrauterine contraceptive (IUD), pain, depression, back problems, vaginal dryness, vaginal douching, or having a new sex partner, it can also be caused in women who are not even sexually active![20] If you develop a bacterial infection of this type while taking Azilect, you may need to be treated with metronidazole (Flagyl), or clindamycin. However, you must be careful because Flagyl may interfere with other PD medications, as well as predispose you to lightheadedness and subsequent falls. Azilect is also known to cause frequent urinary infections, which can make your already troublesome bladder problems worse![21]

Hence, it can be extremely hard to be the sex diva your mate wishes or that you envision when you have constant bladder issues, vaginal irritation, or irregular menses due to Parkinson's.

Bladder Problems in Women with PD

Constant bladder urgency and frequency are very common in PD, particularly as you advance into mid stages and beyond. Frequent bathroom trips make it extremely hard to maintain good hygiene and cause you to more likely contract an infection from public bathrooms, as well as develop a yeast infection similar to a baby's diaper rash (yuck!) from constant wiping and friction. The irritation alone will predispose you to having chronic infections and more susceptible to dryness (independent from dryness caused by medicines and Parkinson's itself), making sexual intercourse painful at times and less desirable even if your own libido is chemically revved up. This dichotomy of mind and body can certainly leave one feeling emotionally drained and somewhat schizophrenic, contributing to feelings of negative self-worth and unattractiveness and not very sexual at times. Be careful not to confuse irritation and burning in your vagina due to infection with sexual desire. It has been known to happen and can only make things a whole lot worse!

So, you seek the help of a team that includes a urologist, gynecologist, and neurologist to feel normal again. You try several medications, which can help, but they, too, can increase urinary infections and dryness. You even do behavioral therapy and consider things like Botox and sacral stimulator implants to correct the urgency, along with multiple medication trials. But in the end, all these options and treatments can wear out the goddess in you that even if your body finally says YES... your MIND says Absolutely NOT! I just need to sleep!

Even at nighttime, the constant up and down of having frequent urination can be so disruptive, leading to poor sleep for you and your mate. The nightly commotion may lead many to seek separate sleeping arrangements, which could draw a wedge in a couple's intimacy if they are not careful.

In my experience, women with PD have bladder issues due to several factors and not always the same each time for the same person. So, maintain a diary of what triggers frequency and urgency—things like caffeine, alcohol, chocolate, or spicy food intake. Find out if it is caused by intercourse or aggravated by constipation, in which the massive extension of the rectum can stimulate the nerves around the pelvic floor and bladder, giving a sense of urgency. Drink lots of water but not after six p.m. if you have nighttime increased urgency, and remember that urine output increases with age at night. You may ask your doctor for estrogen cream to help with dryness and discuss various medical and surgical treatments, as follows: 1) sacral nerve stimulators, 2) Botox A injections, and 3) other more invasive procedures available to help with bladder problems. Also, seek behavioral modification as early as possible from a certified professional.

Behavior modification entails a strict commitment on the part of the patient in order to improve voiding. If done properly, it can be very effective. Insurance will pay for this; however, you must go to a trained professional experienced in this type of therapy to have a greater success rate.

I recommend behavioral training of your bladder in conjunction with other medical treatments. This type of therapy epitomizes "individualized medical care." The program typically includes voiding diaries, timed voiding, pelvic floor muscle strengthening exercises, and urge suppression techniques (e.g., distraction, self-assertions). Additionally, it includes biofeedback, electrical stimulation into sacral nerves or pelvic muscles, fluid management, caffeine reduction, dietary changes, i.e., avoiding bladder irritants like caffeine, chocolate, and spicy foods, to name a few, weight loss, and other lifestyle changes, including Kegel exercises.

Pharmacotherapy includes a number of oral and transdermal (across skin) medications. These can be very effective and used if behavioral therapy failed or in combination. However, their efficacy is limited due to side effects, although usually non-life-threatening. All medications come in extended release. **The medications in this class include:**

- oxybutin (Ditropan, Oxytrol)
- tolterodine (Detrol)
- solifenacin (Vesicare)
- fesoterodine (Toviaz)
- darifenacin (Enablex)
- mirabegron (Myrbetriq)*
- trospium (Sanctura)** *(does not cross blood brain barrier)*.

> * **Mirabegron (Myrbetriq)** is a newcomer for those who cannot tolerate antimuscarinic drugs, i.e., all the drugs I just listed above. Although it may act as one, it is primarily a beta-3 adrenoreceptor. I find this medicine to work very well especially for those women who have mixed type urinary problems- which in my experience is a great number of us- having components of both an overactive bladder as well as an increase in sphincter control causing difficulty voiding and retention and more likely to cause repeated UTIs (urinary tract infections).[22]

> ** **Sanctura** is best suited for treatment of elderly PD patients due to less side effects, particularly that of altered mental status. Typical side effects of this class of drugs include dry mouth, constipation, dyspepsia, urinary retention, urine infections, impaired mental status, and dry and itchy eyes. Since many of these symptoms can already occur with PD or as a side effect of other PD medications, you have to be extra vigilant when starting these meds, and discuss any sudden changes with your physician ASAP!

As a Parkinson's specialist, I have used all of the older medications on all my patients through the years. However, in dealing with my own personal bladder issues along with those of multiple PD women, including those of my grandmother, I realized how much more devastating this problem can be for young women with PD who are trying to lead active, "normal" lives. Having to live a life that revolves around knowing exactly where the bathrooms are at all times or, worse, having to worry about if there will be bathrooms nearby, is no walk in the park for young or old. It is especially difficult for those women who have to self-catheterize. Even if it's with a cute lipstick-looking device, it's never any fun. Self-catheterization even with newer smaller devices still poses a risk for repeated infections and trauma (physical and emotional). Also, the cost can be absolutely devastating, and that is assuming that the rigidity and tremors and all other Parkinson's symptoms allow you to do this successfully each time. Imagine going to the bathroom at least ten times an hour or more? That does not give you time to do anything else and can leave one completely and utterly exhausted, not to mention disheartened. I, too, found myself in this state before. So, I am extremely glad that this latest drug, mirabegron, has surfaced to the market, making a HUGE impact in the lives of many of us women. Parkinson's women were once doomed to self-catheterizing, surgery, repeated Botox injections or keep living life in the shadows. For many, including myself, mirabegron has been a godsend, returning quality of life and renewing hope where once it was lost.

The key when dealing with bladder issues in the female Parkinson's patient is to remember that we are dealing with two very complex systems, which oftentimes function independent of one another. Therefore, I find that most women with PD who have bladder problems usually have a multifactorial amalgam of issues—having an enlarged rectum due to constipation, trouble voiding because they can't move fast enough, or increased frequency due to misfiring of neurons, plus the fact that many of us may already be predisposed to having increased bladder infections just by being women or having stress incontinence due to childbirth. Therefore, I urge you to speak to your neurologist in detail, keep a diary, and seek help from a team of specialists.

Other lifestyle changes that may help you and your partner keep the flame until the right solution for your problem becomes available is sleeping apart, as long as you don't forget to smooch before or after. This way your constant bladder urgency at bedtime will not disrupt your partner's sleep.

Tips to prevent constant irritation and dryness in the vaginal area:

- Don't use vaginal washes or douches.
- Use Desitin or equivalent to prevent essentially a "diaper" rash equivalent from constant wiping. You may even get a compound of triamcinolone and nystatin from your doctor.
- Avoid harsh soaps and perfumed soaps to prevent further irritation in that area.
- Use cotton underwear or at least those with a cotton crotch if you have a tendency to have recurrent infections. If this is the case, also implement vitamin C intake daily, as well as drink two 4 oz. glasses daily of cranberry juice to prevent and also speed up recovery at the beginning of a urinary tract infection.
- Always shower before and after intercourse to prevent bacteria from entering the urethra.
- Always wipe front to back for same reason.

If you happen to be in the majority of women who get recurrent infections from intercourse, try changing positions as this may help reduce friction on your urethra and decrease the risk for infection. However, if you are still an unlucky soul that gets recurrent infections just by the mere mention of sex, then you will most likely benefit from an antibiotic to take immediately after sex to help prevent the likelihood of getting an infection. There are several medicines used for this problem such as nitrofurantoin (Macrodantin) and phenazopyridine (this medication is contained in some over-the-counter drugs like AZO). However, consult your physician always before changing or stopping medications.[23]

Domperidone (Motilium) and PD

Another medication that can wreak havoc with your constitution is domperidone. Although, frequently prescribed for the common GI side effects of PD meds, such as nausea and vomiting, this medication can lead to an irregular menstrual cycle in menstruating women with PD. This may include an increase in bleeding which may lead to anemia and worsen feelings of fatigue, an already common problem in all Parkinson's patients but especially in us women. This may be hard to decipher at first since having PD can alter our menstrual cycle as well. It can also lead to lactation or breast milk production.

Female Cancer and PD

Last, but certainly not least, it is important to note that dopamine agonists and Levodopa have an increased risk for some types of cancer like melanoma, at least twofold, although this type actually is higher in men with PD. Women with PD on the other hand appear to have an increase in breast cancer, although it is still controversial and unclear as to the exact risk.[24] What we do know is that women that have the LRRK2 (leucine-rich repeat kinase 2) gene as a cause of their Parkinson's disease have a higher incidence of breast cancer.[25] If I had known at the time the two were related, I think I would have been so much more aggressive with one of my first female patients with YOPD. Shortly after her PD diagnosis, she was diagnosed with breast cancer. I would have made sure her oncologist was aware of the fact that this was related to her neur logical disease. After her cancer diagnosis, unfortunately, her PD took second stage, but perhaps should have been managed just as aggressively. She will always stand out in my mind as an extremely courageous and brave soul who never faltered in the midst of adversity, dealing with both illnesses. Even as the cancer was winning, she kept a positive outlook and sunny disposition that came from her faith. So now in my quest of educating people about Parkinson's, I must not let the lives of those women who came before me go in vain, but serve as a teaching point to educate other professionals and women who might be at risk about what to look for, since early prevention is always the key to a successful outcome. Therefore, I suggest talking to your doctor about the risk of breast cancer and melanoma, especially with certain PD subtypes. Vigilance is imperative in prevention and early treatment. Together you and your physician can come up with a screening plan appropriate for you and your needs.

- Don't forget to do self-exams routinely.
- Exercise and keep a healthy weight.
- Limit alcohol intake, which will help you sleep better as well.
- Breastfeed if possible.
- Limit menopausal hormone replacement (although some studies show intake of these reduce risk of PD).

Keep a diary of things to discuss when visiting your neurologist—sexual issues, mood swings, headaches, irregular menstrual cycle or worsening PD symptoms with menses to name a few. In this fashion as a true diva you will always be prepared and avoid a "door knob moment" when face to face with your physician. Keep your list to three things so that all issues are fully addressed; if you have more things to discuss, make more frequent appointments. Make sure you prioritize your complaints according to severity of impact on your personal life and that of those around you, especially for those who depend on you.

11

Beauty Tips for the Parkinson's Diva

"Give a girl the right pair of shoes and she will conquer the world!"
~ Marilyn Monroe

Even though I am an absolute shoe fanatic even with PD, all I need is lipstick (a pretty case is nice but Not a must!) and I feel like I can conquer anything! My lipstick and I date back to my years of medical school. Back then, it was a light shade of pink but the feeling was the same.

When I had no time to eat, sleep, or dress in anything other than scrubs, I still would make sure I always had my lipstick case in my white coat pocket. I would always make sure to apply a fresh coat on the way to visit a dying patient, review a challenging case, or when I was on my way to the operating room...as if it would magically give me the strength and will power to take on whatever insurmountable obstacle stood before me.[1] Nowadays, before I tackle the challenges of living with Parkinson's, I still start with a fresh face and a brilliant shade of red—like carrying a cloak of invincibility that requires only a touchup once and again to keep the strength and courage flowing. This seemingly insignificant act of willpower not only says I am still here ready to fight no matter what comes, but also helps me feel "normal" and feminine, and if I manage to accomplish nothing else that day I would at least have exercised my fine motor skills for the day!

I believe this is crucial since the radiance from our faces is one of the most attractive features of a woman. However, I have heard many PD women complain about how they no longer feel attractive as the "mask" takes over or, worse, others begin to judge us as unfriendly or unapproachable, which can add to our inner sadness. Some of us may begin to feel perhaps less capable of facially expressing joys and sorrows in the same fashion as we once were able. They wonder if there is a pill or a shot to reverse this process; after all, there is something magical about a smile that captivates all of our souls, and touches our hearts. A simple smile can infuse passion, desire, and ignite feelings of warmth, love, and happiness in our hearts, even if it comes from a stranger. My daughter once exclaimed spontaneously after a stranger in a passing car smiled at her. "She smiled at me and made my day!" But, as our facial expressions weaken, our smiles seem to fade, contributing to that sense of sadness and dissatisfaction with our lives because our brains typically respond to others by mirroring their expressions. Our long-term facial "flatness" may lead to our own decline in emotional experiences.

Do we smile because we are happy or are we happy because we smile? Putting on my lipstick can make me smile even when I started out not feeling so happy...

So, I think a smile works both ways. We women want to use the power of feeling good about ourselves from an external stimulus to make us smile internally, to keep us from losing our ability to experience emotions. Darwin, too, believed that facial expressions are vital for experiencing emotions. In the "Expression of the Emotions in Man and Animals," he wrote that "The free expression by outward signs of an emotion intensifies it. On the other hand, the repression, as far as this is possible, of all outward signs softens our emotions."[2]. This idea that we must use our facial muscles in order to discern emotion ourselves has been confirmed by studies on BOTOX, which are used on millions of people for cosmetic purposes, usually to get rid of age lines. This medication works essentially by paralyzing the muscles injected—in this case the facial muscle. A study published in Psychological Science journal revealed that having this procedure impaired the individual's ability to process the emotional content of languages; hence, their overall emotional experience. Other scientists have argued that feedback from facial muscles which produce expression are critical in regulating an individual's emotional status and experience.

Hence, the same is presumed to be the case in PD patients suffering from *"masked facies"* which means expressionless facial demeanor. Diminished facial expressivity occurs earlier in the disease and is unrelated to depression[3] Some investigators have also documented this finding of loss or impairment in being able to correctly identify emotional prosody, i.e., word intonation; emotional scenes or faces. However, these findings have not been consistent across all studies, leading some to speculate that findings differences may be related to methodology "On" vs. "Off" state, as well as the presence of other cognitive impairments.[4] Moreover, some researchers have found that PD patients have specific deficits in the process of particular emotions like "fear" and "disgust," compared to other emotions.[5] This finding in my opinion supports what Darwin and studies in Botox have found— that in order to produce appropriate emotional responses we require feedback from our own facial muscles, which mimic or mirror the expressions of others. In the case of fear and disgust, almost the entire face is involved in producing these emotions. Hence, if you can't burrow your frown, raise your eyebrows, or grimace due to rigidity, slowness and weakness, the expression will not be encoded appropriately into your brain.

One of the biggest complaints I hear from women with PD is the fact that they would do anything to be able to have normal facial expression and a normal radiant smile. They often ask me if there is something they can do to improve their "masked faces." After all, our face is what people see first and if we look "unhappy" due to what I discussed above— decreased muscle tone and weakness—others may get the impression that we might not be as friendly or approachable as we really are. The problem magnifies particularly if our voices are also beginning to fade, i.e., hypohonia.

In order to combat the effects of Parkinson's on our bodies, we need a combination of both internal and external stimuli to allow us to be able not only to express ourselves better but read others appropriately. Many PD patients, especially women, tend to suffer from apathy (upwards of 50%) and depression, both known as negative factors. However, one does not necessarily precede or is the cause of the other. But, apathy, lack of initiative and motivation, is more likely with increasing cognitive impairments.[6] Both depression and apathy are inherent parts of the disease, just like tremors, and not an adaptability or coping mechanism problem. So what can you do to help yourself combat these feelings?

- Educate yourself about the disease.
- Take an active role in managing your PD, including talking to your doctors about the feelings of apathy that may color or influence any negative emotional reactions.
- Decrease stress by doing exercises (remember, this increases natural endorphins and is shown to improve depression and cognition), getting involved in church (finding spiritual comfort) or other religious activities, get together with a girlfriend who uplifts you.
- Accept help and ask for help when needed.
- Try to continue your "normal" activities. This may be able to be accomplished to an extent by making some modifications to lifestyle and accepting limitations and embracing new talents and ways of looking at the world, which means wearing some clothes you love, but with some changes such as more zippers or bigger buttons; and great shoes, but lower heels and more rubber slippery soles, etc.
- You may need to alter medications by either increased dose of dopamine, or adding stimulants like Provigil, Adderall, or antidepressants.

So we try our best to feel attractive, interesting, and appealing to others. One way to boost your spirits and have you smiling voluntarily is wearing clothes and accessories that suit your personality. In my opinion, if you laugh a lot, put on makeup, such as lipstick, you will be stimulating the facial muscles externally to maintain your ability to read emotions appropriately, but also internally by producing or releasing both natural dopamine and serotonin because you "feel" good, causing you and others to smile. At the same time, a radiant smile makes any woman look younger and more appealing. Remember, a nice smile is not only contagious but can cure a multitude of ailments. Yes, I believe in the power of red! Without red you can't have REDemption, or be cuRED!

Go ahead, apply your favorite shade today, even if you are not in the mood, and let your face reflect the inner beauty of your soul and work those face muscles daily. Pucker up and kiss someone you love, laugh out loud until you cry, let every muscle of your face be free and express itself. You will be glad you did!

I, like Audrey Hepburn, believe that the *"happy girls are the prettiest girls."*[7]

Therefore, no matter if you are a woman of twenty-five or eighty-five, single, widowed, married, or divorced; you should have your own sense of STYLE that is UNIQUELY yours. I want to encourage all of you to not merely be women of fashion but rather women of style, because fashions are fleeting, but true style is a thing of beauty that endures forever if it comes from within you. Just because we suffer from Parkinson's, does not mean that we women enjoy any less dressing up, looking pretty, and feeling our best. Especially when we are lacking self-esteem or feeling worn down, the compliments of our significant others or the occasional harmless flirtation from a good-looking man can go a long way to lift the spirits. When worn appropriately, clothes can be extremely empowering. Dress the way that makes you feel better; even more, dress as the woman you want to become, a leader, an innovator, a world changer. The key is molding your own brand of style to fit your dreams, ambitions, present roles, careers with your newly or longstanding diagnosis of PD. Dress as the woman you want to become based on a future image of yourself, leaving all past failures and doubt behind only as a reminder of how far you have come.

With a little practice and knowing what to look for, this can be accomplished. Especially since I hear so many women with PD say that since they got diagnosed with the disease they stopped applying makeup, wearing jewelry, doing their nails, or wearing heels; in a word, they stopped being feminine. It's not that we don't want to look pretty, but it is so darn hard to find the right accessories, makeup products, jewelry, shoes, etc. to be able to be comfortable and not risk injuring ourselves like poking an eye out while applying mascara or falling because of the "cute, stylish" shoes, so we go without!

As someone who loves fashion and refuses to let PD rule her life, I am here to assure all of you that fashion and style can be maintained; however, it does require bit more effort to accomplish the desired look. And that extra effort is worth it if it empowers you.

You know that when you look good, you feel good and thus you have more energy. The extra spring in your step will be greatly appreciated by those who depend on you, like your family.

My goal is to have you bring out your own style and personality through your wardrobe, mixing old pieces of clothing with new ones. You do not necessarily have to follow the traditional rule of pastels or floral patterns; in fact, neutral colors may work best for some of you because they can be easily coordinated with new(er) pieces while making your own personal statement. You don't have to spend a lot of money to achieve a chic look! I bet you already have a lot of great pieces in your wardrobe. What you may need is to modify some of those clothing pieces to accommodate your new lifestyle, i.e., changing small buttons for larger ones, replacing buttons with zippers, especially down the front of your sweaters or blouses, or snap buttons (if you have a caregiver, consider placing these snap buttons on the back of your clothes), or even hooks, which I just love. There are so many types and styles of hooks which can lend personality to your garments. Add elastic to skirts and pants or even Velcro to the pants for easy dressing. You may have to buy a couple of pieces that go well with things in your collection that are easy to wear and take off when you are in an "off" state. This also involves rearranging your wardrobe so that all your essentials are at eye level, or waist level at the lowest, because if you are stiff and rigid in the morning as most of us are, you cannot be bending down to look for socks, etc. in the bottom drawer.

Since I was diagnosed with PD, all of my essentials in the kitchen, bathroom, and closet are at eye or waist level since I can no longer climb or bend down. Like me, the first thing you want to reconsider in your wardrobe is the COMFORT and ACCESSIBILITY of your clothing; in other words, ease of getting into clothes. The ability to get in and out of clothes without much effort reigns supreme with all of us women that have Parkinson's. This means wearing clothing that allows us freedom to move with ease, and are comfortable to wear during dyskinetic episodes, made of breathable materials such as cotton, linen, silks, spandex. The added benefit is these materials mix well with Lycra for extra comfort, durability, and softness. These clothes should be practical for those times when your motor function just won't cooperate. A tall order, I know.

Living with PD is already challenging enough without having to struggle with your clothing, too. So, if you can't put it on easily or take it off by yourself, then it's not going to be a good piece of clothing for you to keep. I want you to visualize a world with PD where you are not only feminine, but comfortable, and practical as well without having an entire collection of tracksuits, pure spandex, muumuu dresses, or SWEAT PANTS! Velcro is good, but I don't want you to be known as the Queen of Velcro either. I love acetate pants, which are breezy, flowy, and usually have an elastic waist for easy pull. They also make blouses and skirts of this material—hurray! But my favorite blends are mixture of cotton, polyester, rayon, acetate, and Lyocell with a bit of spandex for everyday wear. The beauty of these mixtures is that they do not wrinkle as much, are machine washable, inexpensive, look and feel great, and move with your body!

Lyocell is a great fabric, not only eco-friendly but extremely absorbent—perfect for those of us who experience excessive sweating due to the effects of PD medications. It is a very soft yet a strong, durable fabric and can provide a great deal of versatility to your wardrobe because it can be made to look like natural products such as leather or silk. I love the feel of cashmere, silk, and satin, but they are more expensive and harder to maintain their look. You should have at least a couple of pants with elastic at the waist, easy to pull on and off for those days when fine motor skills are not at their best, especially if you have a history of bladder problems. Especially in the face of bladder issues or if you need someone to assist you with changing, two-piece garments are much better and easier to maneuver. However, I do caution you to not get too comfortable in stretchy pants. Believe it or not, your family does pay attention to what you wear and how you look, especially if you have children, and even your husband is watching whether he says so or not. It is easy to gain weight if not careful if constantly wearing elastic waist garments. Not long ago, my husband said," I see you are wearing jeans again today! Is it because you know you look good in them?" I had to laugh. "No!" I replied, "It's because our daughter wondered if I owned any other types of pants since I seem to be living in my 'stretchy' pants lately." I had explained to my daughter that my recent fashion faux pas had nothing to do with my sense of style, but more of a practical matter since I had been extremely stiff and barely able to even put on my flexible pants in the morning. This was obviously a sign I needed to increase my medication.

So, just because you wake up frantic, frazzled, and frustrated, there is no reason to look the part, as I have demonstrated above. We all have families, responsibilities, and duties to tend to; therefore, we must put our best foot forward. But, getting started takes a lot of effort and concentration especially if you are shaky, rigid, dystonic, off balance, having freezing spells, or simply dyskinetic. I have been there more than once! BELIEVE YOU ME! Getting ready in the morning is a full-time job all on its own sometimes.

If you are stiff in the morning like I am, get up an hour early to take medications. If it is extremely difficult to get out of bed, keep medications by the bedside to avoid injuring yourself or falling. In this manner by the time you actually have to get going, they will be in your system and you can move without tripping, falling, or dropping things. You will also be more flexible, making it easier to shower, dress, and begin the day's activities. If you take other medications with similar side effects, i.e., that lower blood pressure, or cause drowsiness, such as blood pressure pills, make sure to space out the medications to avoid compounding side effects like a sudden drop of blood pressure, which will then incapacitate you, causing dizziness, sleepiness, and feeling faint.

One of the biggest problems I hear in women with PD is the inability or difficulty with putting on a bra. This is an important first layer, as we often hear in fashion articles or on makeover shows: *the first thing a lady needs is a nice bra to support the girls and make you feel like a sexy woman!* Although there is still a debate today as to whether bras are really needed, I am a firm believer that the "girls" must be properly cuddled and lifted to give us that wonderful feminine silhouette, which adds confidence to our walk and makes all of our clothing look so much better—trust me. If you are having trouble putting on a bra, this tells me that you are most likely under-medicated and need to have your medications either increased or adjusted to improve your stiffness and range of motion and to decrease tremors. However, if increasing your medications does not improve your mobility, your doctor needs to be looking at other causes like nerve impingement in your neck or shoulders that could be preventing this. Either way you must begin with a serious talk with your doctor about this problem, followed by a thorough evaluation, medication adjustment, along with physical therapy to improve range of motion. After evaluation, if the problem is found to be non-reversible, then I suggest various alternatives. However, unless you have small breasts or have always gone "bra-free," I don't really suggest foregoing this essential undergarment. It makes me so sad to hear beautiful, vibrant women with PD give up on wearing bras. Because what I hear is *I am giving up on being a woman and dressing up for the occasion.*

By no longer caring or bothering, we are unwillingly admitting defeat and letting Parkinson's win. What we are essentially telling our brains is that it has no control or power over the situation we are in. But, I am here to say that we as women have many options besides going bare.

There are other alternative garments or ways of putting on a bra that will allow us to look and feel feminine. Options are switching to bras that close in the front. Do the hook-and-spin technique of hooking and front then turning the bra; if you apply talcum makes this process a lot easier. Another option is buying camisoles with built-in bras. Make sure they are made of cotton and comfortable because the PD meds can makes us perspire a bit at times. We want to stay cool and also want to be able to put the cami on with ease, so nothing with spandex here. Also, you can use NuBra, which are adhesive cups you can place on your breast. You can try a bandeau, a strapless bra that covers the breast. Many women with mobility issues have sworn by bandeau bras. Finally, if you must go bra-free, you can wear shirts with front pockets that cover each breast.

The second most commonly talked about problem and frustration in women with PD is not being able to wear certain shoes or heels, particularly if you experience dystonia or foot cramps. I, too, have felt this frustration. Once again, may I remind you that if you are having significant dystonia or cramps interfering with being able to put on shoes, then this is a sign that your medications are not at optimal levels and it needs to be discussed with your physician. In the meantime, I suggest that every woman with PD gets at least one pair of shoes that are a size too big— for those times when your feet or toes cramp; it is easy to slip on an oversized shoe, but it must be a fully closed shoe. I like Dansko clogs for this problem because you don't have to bend or even sit down to put them on; they simply slide on. I also like Clark's shoes due to general comfort and ease in putting on, plus they have lots of new feminine styles to choose from—my favorite if you are a woman on the run. Although I no longer have the luxury of having my brother-in-law mail me whatever I want straight to my office or home, and actually have to trek down to the Galleria in Houston where he works to get my shoes, they are still my favorite. I can get dressy shoes and sporty shoes all in one place, which are easy to walk in, put on, and wear even when I am completely stiff and rigid and have trouble maneuvering. Some of the shoes also come with zippers, which is very convenient.

The heel size of my shoes might have changed some since I got Parkinson's. Long gone are the days I could parade around in stiletto heels; however, the overall look and feel to my shoes has not changed much. I am always searching for one-of-a-kind, cute, feminine, stylish, and of course now, easy to wear and walk in—a hard task but not impossible! I like dainty and practical and everything in between to fit the occasion. You do not have to forgo heels altogether just because you have PD. But you do have to be more conscientious of the type of heel you wear. Certainly, I don't think that the majority of us with PD will be able to walk around on a three-inch heel or higher without risking the chance of falling and breaking something. However, it is possible to wear two-and-a-half-inch heels at times, depending on the shoe. If you are going to buy a heel, make sure it is a wedge or a large block heel with good support both around your ankle and front of your foot so it does not slip out or aggravate dystonia of your toes. I typically wear one-and-a-half-inch heels; if I want to be bold, I go to two and a half inches. However, rarely, I may find a comfortable cute, feminine shoe with good support that has either a solid block heel or a wedge in a three-inch heel for special occasions if I know I will be sitting most of the time. This way I can have my long leg effect!

Since I became a doctor, I realized the importance of owning a good pair of walking shoes and I encourage you to invest in a good pair. In my profession I was on my feet constantly and I did not like tennis shoes or sneakers because they were not stylish for every day, professional wear, but most importantly until that time I had not found a good pair that did not cause knee pain—until one day I was fortunate enough that my brother-in-law at the time worked at a Clark's company and gave me my first pair of Clark's shoes. I did not think they were the most attractive shoes but neither were they the worst; however, they were heavenly on my feet, being an intern on call for fifty plus hours a week. To this day, Clark's shoes have been my go-to brand for everyday wear when I practiced medicine but especially as I developed PD and I began to experience a lot of foot and toe cramps as well as pain in my feet and legs. They are easy for PD women to use; besides, now they have a wide array of styles and colors to select from. I also like Dansko and L'artiste; the latter is great for comfort, easy to put on, and adds a sense of unique style, particularly for those of us who like a touch of the eclectic, accentuated with color and femininity. L'artiste shoes are usually found in boutiques or can be purchased on the Internet shopping network, Overstock.com. They, too, have a wide selection of colors. The clogs by Dansko are especially good for rainy days because of the traction, which helps decrease falls. However, Dansko is not good for those of you experiencing lots of freezing weather because the sole is not very slippery and will aggravate the feeling of being "stuck" to the floor. You should not wear them if you have too much rigidity, particularly in the legs, because they are a heavy shoe. But if you can overcome the rigidity, you a might get a good workout in your gluteal region as well as in the legs, making your legs more beautiful and stronger!

When wearing and picking out shoes, think of the places you will be wearing them as well the condition of your Parkinson's. When walking, don't get in a hurry. Always use safety measures to avoid falling. Take it from me; it is true what they say about an "ounce of prevention . . ." On my birthday a few years ago, we went out to celebrate. Of course, I had to look dashing. Although I was wearing appropriate shoes, a severe thunderstorm came through suddenly, causing a massive power outage, so we decided to leave the restaurant. This restaurant is known for its extremely slippery stairs, so I always take the handicap ramp. On this day, however, my husband had run out to get the car and was parked in front of the restaurant waiting for me to exit as it was pouring. Rather than risk getting even more drenched as I walked out, I thought I would take the stairs. After all, the shortest distance between two points is a straight line! I was carrying our food, which we did not get a chance to eat before the power went out, in one hand and my purse in the other. Since I had my eyes on my husband rather than on the stairs as I should have, as soon as I placed my first step on the stairwell, I slipped and went bouncing down on my bottom hitting every single blessed step. As I tried to catch myself, the contents of my purse flew all over the place while the pasta I was holding in the opposite hand did the same, landing all over me. It was a sight to behold. Thank goodness I was wearing slacks; otherwise I would have had another exhibitionist moment. Now, each time I go to that restaurant, I shake my head, chuckle, and take the handicap route, even on a perfect sunny day.

Remember, you can wear all types of shoes as long as they provide support, are easy to put on, have slippery soles, and a heel not over two inches high, to avoid tripping and balance problems.

I, like you, know how hard it is to get ready in the morning while trying to get kids to school and husband off to work, especially if you don't feel well. The thought of applying makeup may be a bit overwhelming. So, again a lot of us have forgone this uniquely feminine ritual which completes our outward appearance. When we have severe tremors or dyskinesias, this may seem like the last thing we want to do. But, again I say that with a little extra effort, we can enhance our inner beauty and strength. However, even before you decide to put any makeup on, applying hydrating creams, or moisturizers, make sure you take a good look at the person in the mirror and focus on your best features. Is it your eyes? Lips? Or nose perhaps? Be thankful each day for what you have been given, and then do these simple facial exercises daily to strengthen your facial muscles and keep that beautiful smile going and feelings in check. This will help decrease your masked facies.

Facial exercises: You can do these sitting or standing in front of the mirror, slowly while breathing deeply.

- Raise your eyebrows as high as possible and hold for ten seconds.
- Open your mouth as far as possible and stick your tongue out and hold for five seconds.
- Place three center fingers on your cheeks and press firmly down and smile as hard as you can to raise cheek muscles against fingers.
- Pucker your lips out as far as you can into an "o" shape, then change expression into a wide smile. Repeat three times.

- Wiggle nose from side to side.
- Move your chin from one shoulder across chest to the other.
- Exercise your eyes to decrease drooping. Move first to the right, then left, then up, then down, then diagonally in each direction; all positions for five seconds.
- Look at the ceiling and pucker your mouth like you are about to kiss someone; hold for five seconds. Then stick out your tongue ten times while looking at the ceiling. Then return to normal.

These exercises will help strengthen your neck, face, and eyes. Once you have done your exercises, you are ready for some makeup, if you are in the mood . . .

Yes, it is possible to wear makeup even when you have PD. I have looked at various products considering my experience with patients and my own personal experiences. For beautiful lashes during special occasions, I have found Lancôme mascara—motorized—works best to keep the tremors from causing you to poke your eyes out. Also, there is a motorized powder/foundation, which Lancôme used to carry. But there are also many other brands that carry similar motorized products. Although I have used motorized (best for tremors/ dyskinesias) makeup, I prefer mousse foundations, ones that are easily blendable— look on the label for the word blendable. This means that the foundation will apply easily despite your dystonia and tremors. Many cosmetic companies offer this; I prefer L'Oreal brands but there are others that have mousse blush/ foundation. I use both blush and foundation in this type of consistency as it stays on all day despite the perspiration. It is creamy and smooth so it hydrates my face, which is important. Remember, Parkinson's can also affect our skin texture; plus all those meds, lack of sleep, and constipation can wither skin. I also prefer and recommend those that provide the most UV light protection due to our increase in melanoma risk as PD patients independent of skin type. The other thing you can do to dampen tremors while you put on makeup or mascara is to add small, one-pound weights to your wrist. This will lessen the tremors, giving you better control. Aside from DBS that will surely stop tremors, you may talk to your doctor about Botox in your arms to dampen tremors if other solutions, including medication, are not working.

Use an electric toothbrush to brush your teeth; particularly you have severe rigidity, dystonia, or tremors. Use an electric razor to help depilate your legs as well. To keep your feet smooth and soft, use Amope Pedi. This is also motorized. Now you, too, can have beautiful, smooth feet.

Ladies, make sure to keep your faces well hydrated, Use wedges of potatoes or cucumbers for your eyes, and hydrate from inside out. Make sure to eat and drink plenty of fluids; add some cucumber, pineapple, or orange slices to your water, which not only will gives it a refreshing taste but adds a touch of sophistication.

It is true about the saying: "When you look good you feel good, confidence (will shine through in all your) performance(s)." Maria Sharapova should know what she is talking about since not only is she beautiful but also an extremely talented tennis player. She also understood that fashion was a way to communication and expression just as music and art are.[8]

The power of this positive thinking will not only transform your day-to-day life, but also the lives of those around you.

When you feel good about yourself, you exude a positive aura that others around you will want to emulate.

This, in turn, can lead to a chain reaction of happiness that can be passed on to all those who come in contact with you . . .

Putting forth that extra little effort also keeps your brain from deteriorating while forcing you to establish new highways of communication between brain cells, bypassing the old rusty, slow ones!

Hence, increasing your brain and body performance while decreasing your fatigue levels and ALL because you added your own brand of style to Parkinson's—an elegant look, shabby chic, or like me, simply *diva-licious*! My husband likes to call me "Jackie O" in fun. A good set of pearls goes a long way . . .

For women with PD, clasps are a difficult thing to handle. You don't necessarily have to have genuine pearls that cost a fortune to enjoy the beauty—a good set of faux pearls, which come in long strands, easy to put on over your head, or wrap around if need be, or even those that come with a magnetic clasp. You simply can't go wrong with pearls.

You can dress them up or down. I think every woman should have at least one set of pearls in their collection. Usually, the more fatigued I become, the less attractive and less feminine I tend to feel, which if we are not careful can lead us down a slippery slope to emotional exhaustion and hopelessness. Thus, the harder I have to try to overcome this feeling. Positive thoughts and actions always beget more positive thoughts and actions, so the choice is truly ours. But, the actual gesture to overcome this feeling of unworthiness or apathy may seem insurmountable. Yet, the expression can be as simple as putting on some hot lipstick or wearing a nice, bright-colored blouse or jacket . . .

I often find that my dress colors reflect my inner mood. Typically I am a bright, cheery person who wears bright colors but as I have episodes of depression, increased fatigue or apathy, my color palate tends to become more monochromatic, often dressing in shades of gray—be aware of your changes in style that reflect sadness and apathy. Be aware that dark clothes, especially black, can perpetuate that feeling of depression, but you must learn to put a twist of sophistication to it by adding your own beautiful smile. When I find myself gravitating towards these colors, I have to make a mental effort to put on a bright color even if it's just on my lips or nails. Use a quick drying polish as this not only avoids messes due to tremors but is also much easier to remove. Several brands make these. I like OPI rapid dry topcoat because that's all the energy I have at the moment. Of course, if you have some extra cash, consider doing shellac nails which last two to three weeks. Best way to remove nail polish is by using pre-packaged nail polish wipes!

"Be sure to remember that although pastels can attract joy and giddiness, fleeting emotions are pastel seekers because they lift us up even if it is momentarily just long enough for the storm to pass."[9] The simple mental act which leads me to smile even though I am wearing gray means I can't decide if I am truly independent (white) or still fighting for control over this disease (black)[10, 11]. And begins a positive transformation along with the visual reminder of having purposefully added color to my wardrobe serves further to help me smile and be happy. After all, I have just proven I do have control over my situation. As Audrey Hepburn, a diva of style herself, would say, "I believe in manicures . . . lipstick . . . I believe happy women are the prettiest women." So go ahead, show the world your beauty![12] Let your outer beauty match your inner brilliance.

When I feel good about myself, take better care of myself and feel attractive, I am not only conquering my illness but also strengthening my resolve to keep fighting for a better tomorrow. Start singing, smiling, or dancing even when you don't feel like it and soon enough you will.

In short, whatever it is that empowers you and helps you tackle the world head-on, or allows you to take care of yourself and your loved ones, be a better mother, spouse, sister, daughter, Parkinson's advocate; embrace it, and make it a part of your daily routine for the whole of next year and every year! But don't forget to include facial massages, and exercises to keep muscles strong to allow you to continue processing the world around you to the fullest!

Make living with Parkinson's disease a work of art where you are the masterpiece! You can become as one of those precious rare art pieces in the Japanese culture that are repaired with gold to fix small imperfections and cracks, known as the art of kintsugi or kintsukuroi.[13] Japanese believe that when something has suffered damage and has a history, the addition of gold makes it more beautiful, so, too, we who suffer chronic illnesses like Parkinson's become more fragrant and extraordinarily beautiful, which comes from the soul due to having been broken and repaired through the teachings of daily living with PD.

12

Tools & Gadgets Every Parkinson's Diva Should Own

"Do not wait; the time will never be 'just right.' Start where you stand, and work with whatever tools you may have at your command, and better tools will be found as you go along."
~ George Herbert

I am sure you all have experienced the frustration of doing a simple chore like breaking an egg for breakfast, and thirty minutes later having to wipe off counters and floors because you accidentally shattered the egg in your hand because of the rest or action tremors, or because the egg went flying off your hand onto the floor due to the same tremors.

Other times, these pesky oval shape objects just refuse to stay put and simply roll off the counter, but by being too slow to catch them before they reach the ground, all you are left with is a big mess! Or worse, that frustrated feeling of biting into a crunchy egg time and again because much to your chagrin, you accidentally broke the egg into a hundred pieces and could not fish all the shells out from the frying pan while cooking it. Or at least you thought you did.

To avoid making a mess in the kitchen with eggs or having to fish out shells from your scrambled eggs or having to eat crunchy eggs, I suggest investing in an egg cracker. I have found both an egg cracker and an egg cracker/separator on Amazon for just a few dollars.

At other times, the biggest accomplishment for the day, in my case, is sewing a pair of my daughter's favorite, cozy socks. I could not thread the needle due to poor fine motor skills, along with tremors and dystonia, which only made using one of those needles with an open top even more difficult. The constant jerking of my involuntary movements in my hands did not allow me to make more than a couple of stitches at a time as I unwillingly pulled the thread out of the needle the tenth time!

So frustrating I just wanted to scream! Funny thing though, my husband in seeing my desperation thought he would come to my rescue but, alas, to my surprise, he, too, was unable to thread the needle! A sigh of relief on my part, to not feel so completely useless! I was absolutely determined to get my daughter's socks fixed.

Triumph at last! Thirty-five minutes later, I had sewn the darn socks and I was UTTERLY worn out! But I was feeling so very proud of my victory over the needle and thread.

Afterward, I thought to myself, "*There MUST be a better way!*"

I thought I would research the best way to thread a needle for people like me and you. I discovered that you can find needle threaders at Walmart, Hobby Lobby, arts and crafts or sewing places…again, you can have either wooden or metal ones. I prefer the metal ones; the wooden ones may have a better grip, are less likely to slip, and are easier to see. Prices range between $1.50 to $17. I would not spend more than $5.

I began to share my findings with others, which in turn has led to building expertise of what works and does not work for most of us.

In the process I have been collecting gadgets and tools to help make life easier for those living with his/her so-called PD. Plus, my girlfriends are equally awesome because each time they see some cool gadget that appears practical BUT feminine and worthy of a diva, they buy it for me to try. Recently, they bought me a set of beautiful wine goblets that look like the real thing except they are plastic and even have some sparkle—just a little, not too much. I don't want to stop traffic or blind someone!

So if I drop them, I won't be breaking any more dishes hopefully. Because I have broken so many good dishes it is not even funny, most have been replaced with attractive, durable, plastic dishes.

Of course, all of you know that opening a jar is almost impossible. One of my dear friends got me a can/jar opener that serves as a bottle opener that adjusts to all different sizes; the beauty of it is that it is hard plastic. The best part of it is that it is extremely feminine with royal blue and white polka dot print. You can have your very own, which also comes in red, on the QVC shopping network. No kitchen should be without one of these fancy, feminine "grippers" which will make your kitchen pop with color while allowing you to open bottles and jars with ease. If this sounds too fancy for your taste, you may still find some old rubber grippers lying around that were distributed by Novartis Pharmaceuticals, makers of Stalevo, a few years ago. Ask your doctor if they have any lying around. If you are not particularly fond of the "fancy" stuff, I found some rubber grippers to open jars just like the one I got from Novartis for as low as $3.99.

These can open bottles, jars, and pill bottles! But I prefer my colorful one, which makes me smile and reminds me of who I am—a total diva even in midst of PD!

Another thing I despise is to wake up discombobulated. The first thing that happens is I spill all my medicines all over the bathroom floor and all I can do is stare idly at my work of art because I am unable to bend down till my medicines kick in, but then again they are on the floor!!! Instead of crying and hiding under your sheets, get a gripper, put tape on the end of it, and pick them up that way, or just grip them one at a time, which may take longer! Speaking of pills, packing medications is the biggest chore I have encountered when going anywhere out of town, even if it's just for a day. Trying to organize all my medications takes me longer than the actual packing of clothes for the trip. Fortunately, I have found a nice pillbox with a zipper from Vera Bradley, which is not only pretty but extremely practical, even for day-to-day managing of medicines.

Just like my bathroom and closet, my kitchen is organized so that all important utensils and tools are easily accessible at eye or waist level, to avoid falling from climbing stairs or getting on the floor and not being able to get up without assistance. Keep a small stepladder with side handles to avoid falls. However, I would not recommend climbing if you have problems, unless someone is there to supervise!

The kitchen can be a treacherous place to navigate. First, if you have decreased sense of smell or no smell, you may be at danger of gas leaks, burning foods, and other potential hazards. So, do install smoke detectors and carbon monoxide (CO) detectors and keep a fire extinguisher handy and up to date. Always double-check the stove or oven when cooking to make sure it has been turned off. Look closely at food expiration to avoid food poisoning.

Then come the actual cabinets, drawers, faucets, cooking items which may make you feel like you are part of the "Beauty and the Beast" scene when all the kitchen utensils attack! Don't sweat the small stuff . . .

Before I became ill, I already had some notion of what was important for making Parkinson's life easier from being a PD doctor for many years. When I designed my office I made sure I incorporated some of the ideas I will discuss here in this chapter. I made sure that my architect knew the importance of gait difficulties that my patients encountered, which included hesitation, festinating, freezing, instability, and balance issues. I asked him to make a flow pattern design for my patients to follow from the entrance to the checkpoint and to every room, not only with a gradual varying color scheme but also in a path they could follow visually. I made sure that the tile on the floor was not too slippery but with enough traction for patients to ambulate with ease. An open space easy to navigate was also paramount. These concepts should also be kept in mind when remodeling or designing your home to be Parkinson's friendly. Now that I no longer practice neurology, I have teamed up with my friend and architect to help design a Parkinson's friendly home from the ground up for a dear friend.

Kitchen[1]

- Replace cabinet handles with long cabinet handles to make opening and closing of cabinets and cupboards easier.
- Install sliding drawers to store commonly used items to avoid needing to reach or bend over to look for things in the back. I had these in my office and they were awesome. I am in process of installing them in my home since I can't climb and I can't easily bend now. Subsequently, all the cabinets in my kitchen at eye and waist level are stuffed to the rim. I am one to decorate for every season but this past Easter I was late in doing so because I had surgery during Christmas and my husband and daughter took off all decorations and put everything on high shelves. When my mother came to visit, she made a point that I did not have my usual decorations out, nor was I in season; I had to explain that I had not been able to do so because everything was too high and I could not climb. That problem was remedied instantly because no diva should have a barren home devoid of pretty vases and things, which make it truly hers!
- Place commonly used cooking items like spices near the stove. I have mine in a drawer next to the stove, which is so very convenient and easily accessible, plus having to avoid bending, stretching, or possible burning if they are above the stove.
- Use a long-handle reacher for lightweight items on high shelves.

Bathroom *(some of same ideas as the kitchen are incorporated)*

- Replace cabinet handles with long cabinet handles to make opening and closing of cabinets and medicine cabinets easier.
- Install sliding drawers to store commonly used items to avoid needing to reach or bend over to look for things in the back. This gives you a great view of all of your medications since on average PD patients take about nineteen pills a day! (Wow!)
- Use a long-handle reacher for lightweight items on high shelves.

- Dressing can be easier if you have a small bench in your dressing area on which to sit.
- I would also invest a few dollars in a reach stick to help pull your pants/undergarments up or other things that may fall.
- Get bars installed in bathtub, by toilet, or in shower if needed to avoid falls.
- Get a shower chair, especially if having difficulty standing or if you have orthostatic/low blood pressure.
- Get a shower extender.

Bedroom: Every Goddess's Inner Sanctum

This should be a sanctuary of peace and comfort with soothing colors to help rest, and decluttered to avoid falls. No bright lights on clocks, no noisy wall clocks, no TVs, and no computers to help you sleep at night! Finding the right color is crucial because color is what will set the rhythm and mood of this space. This is the one space where you have to be most honest with who you are and be true to yourself, so pick a color that represents your personality. But, think also of our main goal of creating a tranquil environment for you to retreat from the stresses of life, PD, and to be able to get a good night's rest. Keep in mind the following when choosing the right color scheme:

- **Blue**   Associated with tranquility; promotes emotional depth and love.
- **Yellow** Fun, uplifting, and encourages humor, logic, and intellect.
- **Red**   Known for its relation to passion, stamina, increased energy, and spontaneity.
- **Green**   Symbolizes acceptance, balance, harmony, love, and communication.
- **Orange** Promotes creativity, productivity, optimism, and enthusiasm.
- **Violet**   Also promotes artistic creativity, imagination, and meditation.

- **Brown** Associated with wholesome, earthly things, creating a safe haven, common sense.[2, 3]

After you successfully transform your bedroom by picking the right color, you must also consider your bed. Since being able to rest and get a good night's sleep is of the utmost importance to look and feel our best, what we sleep on matters. Of course, a nice plush mattress will do us all good but I am talking about considering the thickness of the mattress, not just for comfort but also for practical purposes. After all, for many of us our mobility tends to be worse at night and in the mornings as our medicines are just kicking in or wearing off, making getting in and out of bed difficult if the bed is too low to the ground. It is easier to sit and lie down and much easier to climb out of a bed when you are stiff if doing it out of a taller, i.e., higher bed, one where you are almost standing up when you sit in bed! Trust me, it is a lot easier to get up and out from a bed that is elevated when you are stiff than from one that has a standard mattress size at standard floor level. Having a low bed will make you more prone to fall and injure yourself.

If you are experiencing alterations in blood pressure, especially if having orthostatic episodes, it would be best to have an adjustable bed or mattress so that you might be able to control the angle at which you recline. In this case, you want to maintain the head of the bed elevated at a forty-five degree angle at night because this is when blood pressure goes up and people are more likely to have strokes—in this case a higher risk of intracerebral hemorrhage from a sudden elevated blood pressure. On the other hand, if it gets too low, it is easy to elevate the legs and recline the head down to increase blood circulation to head. The other advantage of having an adjustable bed is that according to some of my previous patients and their bed partners, this is an excellent choice for those that have rapid eye movement (REM) sleep behavior disorder, or restless leg syndrome (RLS). The continued movement of the Parkinson's patient does not easily transmit to the other side, allowing the spouse or bed partner to sleep with fewer interruptions. You may even buy a separate temperature control that can be added to your bed or to the adjustable bed to help with those night sweats we all seem to have due to levodopa compounds. Finally, if you have to purchase any equipment, even a bed, due to specific requirements due to your illness, have your doctor write you a prescription for that object including diagnosis, which will help you save money.

By making these few modifications to your home and lifestyle, you can avoid falls, cut down on frustration, fatigue, dressing time, and cooking time.

Feeding Utensils

I love seafood and have come to the realization that I have increasingly more difficulty eating the shellfish I love unless someone helps me crack the shells, etc., particularly when I am very rigid and slow. Good luck! I have had my own Julia Roberts scene of making shellfish fly across the room once, landing on the head of a woman sitting across from us! It was quite hilarious and embarrassing at the same time. My husband commented why was I throwing away the expensive seafood and not the rice, which was cheap? I said because rice is sticky but when we got up to leave, lo and behold, I had a nice decorative trim on both my pant legs at the hemline made of rice! Now I only order crab or lobster if someone else, like my husband, can take it out of shell for me; otherwise, I order dishes where the shell has been pre-removed.

Sometimes using spoons can be a challenge, especially if I am very shaky! Fortunately, now they have several spoon models to choose from to accommodate your taste and needs. 1) weighted spoon; 2) swivel spoon; 3) long handle spoon; 4) vibrating spoon, a spoon that shakes to counteract hand tremors—Litware device with no "on" switches to fumble with. Major drawback is the price of $300 via Amazon or other companies' websites and not covered by Medicare or insurance! This is a great gift if you have the extra money, and especially useful for those who have both an action tremor component as well as rest tremor, because as you may recall, Parkinson's tremors are purely at rest, which means that when you begin to perform a voluntary action, tremors will cease by definition![4]

Another way you can dampen the tremors is by buying small wrist weights, one-half to one-pound weights, and strapping on at time of eating. You can purchase these weights in places like Academy Sports. This latter can also help you drink better without spilling. But if weights are not enough, consider use of cups with lids, cups with rotating handles, or the tri-stand cup.

Grooming/Bath Products

Grooming sometimes can be challenging especially if you live alone and/or are getting into middle and advanced stage of the disease. So, I recommend keeping these following products handy: a long shoe horn, Velcro or snap buttons to replace ordinary buttons, a device similar to a needle threader that an occupational therapist can provide to help button smaller buttons or zip up pants, and a grab stick to help pull your clothes up. I personally have trouble wearing boots now if they don't have a zipper but even if I manage to get them off, I can't take them off without assistance from my daughter or husband unless I use a boot jack (boot remover), which by the way is very handy in helping remove other shoes as well. Just because I have Parkinson's does not mean I have to stop wearing my favorite boots and neither should you! You may find a relatively good economical one on Amazon for under $12.

Other essentials for grooming which every diva should have or at least consider having is a collection of Hydra Shower Burst which comes in various flavors/scents to help relieve stress and anxiety in your daily routine via a combination of aromatherapy and hydrotherapy. The scent is released as you shower. Most scents are a combination of lavender, which is known to lower heart rate and blood pressure and thus put you in a calm state.[5] Now, combine this effect with water therapy (hydrotherapy) which for centuries has been used by humans as a holistic treatment to balance the mind and body.[6] Hippocrates, the same one we doctors get our Hippocratic Oath from, saw water therapy as having power to get rid of lassitude, i.e., mental and physical weaknesses. Two thousand years later, medical scientists still believe in the healing power of water because it helps to decrease cortisol, a stress hormone, and help to balance or restore the "feel good" neurotransmitter, serotonin.[7, 8, 9] After treatment like this, you will soon be on your way to finding your inner diva and ready to face the world. Best of all, it is a very affordable treatment you can do in the comfort of your home or take with you when you travel.

There are other products that would come in handy in bathing or shampooing if you are having a bad/off day, convalescing from another illness, taking care of a bedbound or decreased mobility loved one, or simply too cold to get wet! A little cold hydrotherapy can do wonders for the soul and body. These dry shampoo products have been gaining popularity since the 1970s, and believe me, they have been a lifesaver many times while I took care of my grandmother with Parkinson's when she became bedbound. Many of my long-standing hospitalized patients' families have also found them useful.

Most of these items can be purchased through the Internet on Amazon or other such sites without having to track out in the cold weather if that would be the case and avoid exposure to the flu/cold during the winter months. A lot of them are also available at any of the local pharmacies like Walgreens.

You may enjoy a full body wash without water as well as shampoo your hair by using a dry shampoo. This could be particularly beneficial if recovering from any other medical illness, especially an upper respiratory one. Other times you may simply be too debilitated to take a shower or bath on your own, such as when you just gave birth to a baby and are still recovering from the PD symptoms exacerbation or worsening.

List of Some Dry Shampoos
- Fresh Start Waterless Foam by TREsemme
- Rub-Out Dry Cleanser by Ojan (with extra thirty seconds, get a scalp massage!)
- Rene Furterer Naturia Dry Shampoo (peppermint adds lift and body to hair)
- Oscar Blondi Pronto Dry Shampoo Spray (fresh, just-washed scent)

- Clean Dry Shampoo by Sephora (clean linen fragrance, time-released, all-day enjoyment of feeling clean)

Do not spray too close to scalp. For best results spray at least six inches away and let set for two minutes. Do not blow dry or comb. Use both on roots and ends. Powder vs. spray powder is best for people who are sensitive to odors and pesticides; it soaks oils and odor best, leaving no odor behind. If you need to reach for dry shampoo a third time, it is time to go the traditional route!

You can also purchase a "No Rinse Body Wash" for $7 if you like. This works best if allowed to lather up and then towel dry. The good part is that it is odorless and hypoallergenic. It contains no alcohol, which is ideal for hospital or convalescing patients. These can be purchased over the counter at any drug store.

You can buy several brands of dry shampoo or Cleanis Aqua Shampoo Gloves. I recommend you use one glove for short or medium hair and two for long hair. This product comes in a package of 12 for $10.

Furthermore, if you have trouble washing because of rigidity, tremors, and/or dyskinesias, I recommend purchasing a bath kit that includes brushes and foot brushes with extra-long handles to allow you to wash without bending, twisting, or reaching. This kit is perfect for those of us with limited mobility and can be purchased for $20. Alternatively, you can buy just a Body Care Long Handle Body Washer alone at a cost of $16.

Lastly, you may also find a no-rinse shampoo cap for $5.

There are so many products to choose from. Basically, it's just finding one that meets your needs and works with your type of hair and body condition. You can also find similar products for "dry" body wash. These can usually be found at a pharmacy over the counter. These products came in handy when I was caring for my grandmother who had PD. Since she was bedbound, all her baths had to be in the bed. Most of the time we used regular shampoo and body wash; however, on those days when she was particularly sick or I was extremely busy, using these fast and convenient products got us through the binds effectively.

Every woman likes to wrap herself in a nice comfortable robe after a bath or shower. But, if you have trouble drying yourself, wrapping yourself in a towel, or putting on a robe, you may want to look into purchasing a towel/cape with Velcro, which makes drying a lot easier.

Medication Organizers

Since we take so many medications and have such busy lives, download an app that reminds you when to take your medicines. (See the iPhone apps section below.) Keep medicines organized in a pillbox. Carry a small pillbox in your purse or on your person along with a medication list so that you are never caught without medications. I personally like the Vera Bradley pillbox, which is not only feminine, pretty, and practical, and you will never lose your pills because your box opened since it has a zipper. It is great for everyday use and for travel, and can hold medications for a little over a week depending how many pills you take. I take close to twenty-three pills a day!

Have a cane handy at all times; you never know when you may suddenly need one like on rainy days, for example, to avoid falls.

Driving Aids[(10)]

If you are still driving or have questions about whether you should be driving, look into getting some GARAGE PARKING AIDS. If you have a problem with vision like I do when my medicine wears out. Vision problems in PD are more common than previously thought. Until I developed PD, I was trained that PD did not affect vision unless you had PSP. So, before you go painting your garage walls neon orange to serve as a visual aid, you may want to try some simple, inexpensive aids which can be found at any local hardware store like Lowe's or Home Depot. Of course this is after you consult your physician to make sure the visual problems are Parkinson's related and appropriate treatment instituted. However, if you continue to have problems, and prisms along with medicines do not correct the problem entirely but you are STILL SAFE to DRIVE, in order to avoid some mishaps in and around your home, look at things like a "parking target." You simply pull up to the stop and when the tire bumps it softly you know you are on target. However, if you have small spaces, this may be in the way and be a higher risk for you to fall if already unsteady and at high risk for falls. Another aid, which might be even more fun, is the flashing LED parking signal. The red stop sign actually flashes LED lights as your car gently bumps into the stick on which it is mounted. It is easy to move out of the way if need be, and reinstall. You can also get a Park Right Garage Laser Park System by Maxsa Innovations, which you mount to the ceiling wall and is triggered by a motion detector that shines light into your car at a predetermined spot. This is one of the best parking garage aids.

Also important is driving a car that fits you. What I mean is that as we become shakier, stiffer, and slower we need to adjust our vehicle to compensate for these problems so that we remain safe on the road. Because all of us with PD have a great deal of fatigue and pain, make sure that you consider ergonomics designed features to help you reduce fatigue, discomfort, such as seats that adjust in at least three directions, and adjustable pedals. Look for comfort, which takes into account ease of entry and exit, legroom, size of control buttons, and voice-activated to recognize your own dystonic, shaky voice so you don't have to fumble with buttons. Also, because we have reduced mobility in our necks, consider one that has sensors in the mirrors to alert you of cars in blind spot or next to you. Also, consider cars that have an automatic parking or park assist. I keep arguing with mine because it is constantly asking me if I need help in parking. I guess I do! Because we have slow reactivity, make sure it does have sensors to stop automatically when something is near. Back cameras are also important. Finally, even the safest of drivers among us can stand some refresher courses from time to time to improve safety. Thus, I recommend that you have a yearly Interactive Driving Evaluation,[11] which can be found at www.SeniorDriving.AAA.com. It takes about forty-five minutes to complete online. It will give you feedback in areas that are needed to address driving risks and how to reduce same. This will also be a good guide for you and your family on points to discuss with your physician, and when a more comprehensive testing is required by an occupational therapist to evaluate your driving and/or when retaking a driving test. This test, which is provided by the AAA, covers five essential areas that are affected by PD:

- Leg strength and overall mobility.
- Head and neck flexibility.
- Low- and high-contrast visual acuity.
- Working memory.
- Visual information processing.

Make sure you are discussing driving issues at least once a year with your physician, or more often if there are changes in your condition, including other illnesses, change in medications, change in mental status, or any other problems that could potentially impair your driving safety.

iPhone Apps[12]

Finally, if you can't live without your smartphone or iPad, there are a few great apps, most of which are free or at a very reasonable price to help make living with Parkinson's a little easier while keeping your busy schedule as a cosmopolitan diva on the go.

One of my favorite apps is called PD LIFE. This app is not only free, but it will help those who need assistance in managing their Parkinson's symptoms by allowing you to record your medications, remind you to take your medicines, and helps to track "on" and "off" states. It is particularly helpful in remembering all the salient issues when you visit your physician. Personally, I give it five high stars.

Next is PatchMate. This app is also free and is great for those of us that are on Neupro patch and have a hard time remembering where they have placed their patches previously? It not only gives you all eight locations but you can also make notes to yourself. It was created by Novartis and is very useful. I give this app four stars.

Lift Stride is another very unique and useful FREE app, particularly for those of us who are already beginning to have gait difficulties. But, even if you are in the early stage, it is never too late to improve your stride. You can do this by walking regularly or by the help of this app. I give it four stars.

Parkinson's Central: If you have to keep up to date with current treatments, caregiving, and research information, this is the app for you—also FREE from NPF. The only downside is that the buttons may be too small for some to use but the bright icons make it easy to navigate. This app gets four stars from me.

Another must-have app is called Life Vac. This app is intended to save a person's life from choking and is especially good for those having swallowing difficulty. The cost is $70. You would need to learn how to use it prior to an emergency. DO NOT learn during an emergency! Would recommend it for caregivers of PD patients but it needs to be used only after receiving appropriate CPR training and ACLS (Advanced Cardiovascular Life Support). The caregiver needs to discuss with the patient's physician for further instructions and recommendations. I give this app three and a half stars because of training required and need strength.[13]

13

Domestic Diva and PD

"The word Diva to me means doing something supernatural with something natural."
~ Patti Lupone, lifehack quotes

As I said before, in order to not only survive PD but to make the best of it, you must start with a positive attitude even when things are shaking all around you. You have to mentally decide to seize the day and make the best of it the DIVA way! This entails doing things in a grand gesture and putting flair to everything you do. This is akin to living loud, which means exaggerating your movements on purpose to trick your brain and awake it from a "slow" mode or bradykinesia. We have Lee Silverman's voice treatment called LSVT LOUD and we have the LSVT BIG physical treatment program designed to improve cognitive skills, function in activities of daily living, ADLs, and decrease movement deterioration by teaching patients to exaggerate movements so they appear normal!

Well, have you ever seen a diva take over a stage or walk down the street? They have purposeful deliberate movements to attract attention, but in our case we want to use this type of mannerism to make our daily functioning appear normal. So, go ahead and sing at the top of your lungs while you are preparing meals or doing house chores; practice voice modulation. It turns out that music releases a large amount of dopamine, making music a great therapy for our disease.[1]

Thus, I highly recommend that you take both music therapy programs as well as the LSVT program. The LSVT program requires a certified speech therapist. Participating in this program usually requires about a month's commitment but is well worth your time, I guarantee it. The earlier in your disease that you begin these programs, the maximum benefit you will receive. Then, practice at home and with friends, or better yet, join a choir or start your own Parkinson's choir. Several Parkinson's groups around the country and world are having great success with this program. One is the "Voces Unidas" led by Claudia Martinez, Hispanic outreach coordinator of the Muhammad Ali Parkinson Center (MAPC) in Phoenix, Arizona for Hispanic Parkinson's patients. Another one is in Spokane, Washington, called "Tremble Clefs."

Invite a group of girlfriends out for cup of coffee and girl talk, especially in loud places, so you have to almost scream. Or have them over to your house for a gathering and play some French or Italian music in the background or whatever music calls to you, so again you have to talk over the music to exercise your voice. Start a book club.

Put a little twist into your cooking or cleaning. Music in the background helps you move faster, especially something with lots of rhythm and beat. Don't worry if you stumble; make it a part of the dance and keep going. Because I can't keep the rhythm for very long, I call my dancing The Parkie Diva Dance. This always amuses my daughter and family tremendously, and it so happens that because I won't let PD dictate my life, I got the privilege of dancing with my dad the last dance of his life! We were both slow and out of *rhythm*, yet it was the best memory I will have for the rest of my life.

My cooking skills have been gradually evolving, thanks to Parkinson's and my grandmother, whose hallucinations include cooking. She would lie in her bed thinking she was baking and making tamales, preparing large meals and so on. She would even say, "Can you smell that? I think the cake is almost done. Can you take it out for me?" What would invariably happen is, when I got home from work, she would ask me to feed her what she had prepared, forcing me to start learning to create those dishes she was preparing in her mind just to keep her happy. However, there were times when she would "make" complicated things, such as tamales, and I would have to go down to the store and buy some pre-made. Sometimes, things did not taste so well and she would let me know—to which I would reply, "Well, grandma, I guess you left it in too long or forgot an ingredient." Then we would both agree that she would do better next time. This was a motivation and incentive for me to get things right. It was always very nice to hear that "her food," essentially my cooking, had turned out delicious. This was a high compliment because she was an excellent cook all of her life.

Over the years, I have become quite the connoisseur of fine cuisine. However, I cannot deny that food simply tastes so much better when someone else prepares it! But I knew I was doing something right when my nephew recently compared my cooking to being almost at the same level as my brother, who is a great cook and aspiring chef!

I also truly enjoy having a tidy home, but I get bored easily with this type of activity and need intellectual stimulation usually outside of the home, which explains my career choice.

However, since I got sick and had to stop working due to PD, I did feel an inner pressure to become more domesticated in order to provide for my family, especially my daughter, in a more consistent manner since I was home. But it was as if there was an expected unspoken rule which dictated that I MUST be able to cook three meals a day, clean, wash, etc., or at least pretend to do all these things!

This was something I had to get used to because when I worked, whoever got home early did the cooking. As far as chores, they were also divided equally, depending on who was off work. This rearrangement of roles and shift in roles can be very difficult for a lot of people when they are used to having things one way and suddenly they are faced with not only having to deal with the blow of a chronic illness like PD, while their world goes topsy turvy in relation to responsibilities in and out of the house. The roles we have played for years or assumed are often intrinsically tied into our personalities and how we view ourselves. For me, being a doctor was more than a profession; it was my identity, which was difficult to separate. At first I was one and the same. After PD, not only did I have to learn to embrace PD, but also embrace myself outside of the medical profession as a vibrant, thriving woman still full of life, dreams, and goals, who just happened to have PD.

I realized that sometimes our lives are interrupted when we least expect it and we feel like we are suddenly thrust into a new path, which we did not want or ask for, and many of us fight it, which causes great tension, discontent, and bitterness. However, sometimes we have to look at it as a new chance to reinvent ourselves and start over as a second chance, if you will! This is a great gift few of us are ever given.

It is not always easy but the journey can be more rewarding and unexpectedly more fulfilling than we ever would have imagined. Thus, I decided to try my hand at becoming the best domestic diva I could possibly be. Mind you, I am and will always be a doctor at heart.

I attempted to learn how to quilt my first year out as a woman with PD, as part of the Parkinson's quilt project for Parkinson's Disease Foundation. I submitted one panel in honor of my grandmother who had PD. She would have been tickled to know: 1) that her granddaughter actually attempted sewing since she and my mom were and are the seamstresses in the family, and 2) that her picture made it all the way to Glasgow, Scotland and Montreal, Canada, since she loved traveling as much as I do but never got the chance to go abroad. I got great help and tutelage from my friend Pat whose mom had been one of my Parkinson's patients. Even though I quilted it for my grandmother, it was in loving memory of her and all my other female Parkinson's patients who had gone before me.

Next, I began to slowly express myself through cooking. I thought that after so many years of marriage it would be nice to put to use all the wonderful cookbooks I was given as a wedding gift, along with the vast spice collection I have accumulated over the years. Losing my smell, as many of you can attest to, makes food tastes blend because smell is an intrinsic part of what makes food taste good. But using the right combination of spices can bring out the flavor even if you can't smell too well. I believe this has been the key to my successful cooking—as per my family. Maybe a little bit of spice and everything nice; in this case, a lot of spice does go a long way. One way to combat the loss of smell commonly seen in PD and other neurodegenerative diseases, such as Alzheimer's, is to engage your entire palate and make it vibrate, thus stimulating taste. Since our tongue only detects four basic tastes, which are bitter, salty, sour, and sweet, by eating spicy, crunchy, aromatic herbs and adding color to your plate, you can engage your other senses, such as sight, to make your entire mouth titillate with joy. Whenever possible add olive oil, butter, roasted nuts, cheese, bacon bits, cranberries, or raisins to name a few.

Avoid combination dishes like casseroles because they tend to hide their individual flavors and dilute taste further.

Salty foods and sweets can greatly enhance the palate but they may not always be medically safe to consume on a regular basis if battling underlying high blood pressure (hypertension), or high blood sugars (diabetes). Always discuss any changes to your diet with your physician.

I personally recommend Cobb salads because of all the different textures. For instance, ham is salty, egg is soft, and croutons are crunchy; better if they are jalapeno-infused for extra kick. Add a bit of roasted nuts, cranberries, or raisins and not only do you have a colorful, flavorful meal, but it is full of antioxidants and nutrients to stimulate the brain. However, you may want to eat this type of food only once a week and eat early in the day; it can slow the digestive tract further because the cellulose in the lettuce is hard to digest.

But as I said before, I can't live in the kitchen even if I wanted to. This so-called Parkinson's disease can make things a bit difficult in the cooking department, not only because of tremors, stiffness, poor coordination, dyskinesias, fatigue, and pain, but also because we may also be caregivers for other sicker, frailer individuals, leaving us with little or no time to go grocery shopping or prepare meals. This is where my other wedding gift has come in handy and has become a must in every Parkinson's woman's kitchen—a crockpot! I highly recommend getting the cookbook called

"Anybody Can Cook in a Crockpot" by Debbie Thornton. This author, who has published several other wonderful cookbooks, is no stranger to Parkinson's herself, since one of her close relatives has suffered from this disease.

When you feel well, I suggest that you prepare large meals and freeze them for those times when you are either too sick or too busy to cook.

It is nice to know that, at least in my daughter's eyes, I have reached Kitchen Diva status. As she dreams out loud about my delicious Thanksgiving meal with my special "pineapple and ginger" sauce, she secretly prays for November to get here soon so she can have her favorite meal, which she will drench in sauce 'specially prepared by her mother.

14

What Every Woman with Parkinson's Should Have

"All you need in life is a friend who has chocolate."
~ Sophie Diehl

First and foremost, every one of us needs a best friend to cry, laugh, and eat chocolate with. Dark chocolate is the best for the brain because it is full of flavonoids and the cacao extract helps prevent memory loss, plus it is a great natural source of dopamine. So, you get to have your Godiva white chocolatini, (this is the only time I prefer white over dark!) keep your brain cells, and bond with your girlfriend, all at the same time. What else can you ask for? Life does not get much better than this. Then again, the unconditional love of a friend who is totally devoted and genuinely invested in your wellbeing, always rooting for you even in the face of adversity, cannot easily be replaced. Such an amazing friend would have no problem dropping everything at a moment's notice to come to your rescue in case of an emergency. For instance, if today happens to be one of those days you simply cannot drive, she would not mind and, in fact, look forward to an opportunity to spending time together and helping out with shopping, cooking, picking up children from school, or even driving you to the doctor three hours away! In fact, these godsend individuals are able to lift you up even without you asking for help. I am extremely fortunate to have such friends. One such friend is Marjie, who became my friend after I took care of her mom with

Parkinson's for many years, and who actually was present when the idea of the Parkinson's Diva was conceived.

I was recovering from surgery with a horrible infection, unable to drive, and stuck at home. On the phone a few days earlier, I told my friend Marjie that it made me sad to hear of women with PD feeling like they were no longer attractive or had lost something in the process and no longer wanting to take care of themselves. I told her, "You know me, as long as I can put on my beautiful high heels and look at them while I am convalescing, I am quite content counting days to be set free again. You know, if I had a tiara and feathers, I would be wearing them right now to speed up my recovery!"

So a few days later my sweet friend pays me a surprise visit with a tiara, feathers, and champagne glasses in hand. We had a blast that day, which extended to my daughter, her friend, and her friend's mom, who had picked up my child from school. It was as if we had gone to a princess makeover party right at home instead of having to travel all the way to Disney World. We danced and laughed so much that my daughter thought we should have more of these parties.

However, I would never have survived thus far without Janet's constant encouragement and support. Having a husband who has had Parkinson's for over fifteen years, she is well versed with all that is Parkinson's and she is an absolute gem! Funny, she and I became friends because I was her husband's PD doctor.

Another wonderful friend who is a diva in her own right is my dearest, oldest, and closest friend Pati. We have known each other for over thirty years, been there for each other's happy times and sad times, and although we don't get to see one another as much anymore because of distance, we remain as close as ever. She remains my sounding board for anytime life decides to throw curve balls at me. We laugh, cry, and draw strength from one another as we always have in the past. There are many other great women in my circle of friends whose support, friendship, and love I cherish dearly and without whose constant support I would not be able to sit here writing this book, because it truly takes a community to care for a chronically ill person.

Without wonderful, selfless people like my friends Irma, Pati, Janet, Lori, Wilma, Johanna, and Nellie, who are not only my biggest supporters and cheerleaders, but also my sounding boards. These precious women have made a real commitment to share the PD journey with me. Because of their unconditional friendship, the treacherous and challenging road ahead does not seem so difficult to travel. They not only challenge and feed my soul, but also stimulate my mind to keep striving for excellence, since each one of them is an extremely accomplished woman in her own right. I would never be able to repay each one for their kindness, generosity, and overall awesomeness, but by helping others who are in the same situation as I am, the love can keep moving forward, healing people and restoring hope to those who seem to have lost their way. Thus, the circle of love can be completed.

When I first got diagnosed, my friend Janet became my right hand for driving because for a while I was completely incapacitated, unable to barely sit up.

Once I began driving, my vision was still giving me problems due to the Parkinson's. I was unable to track the periphery very well, mimicking a peripheral visual field deficit to the point of jamming my car into the left side of the garage on a frequent basis. This was happening so often that my husband started threatening me with buying me a "smart" car to compensate for my "not so smart" driving abilities. At that time I saw a "Hello Kitty" smart car, so I jokingly told him that if I were to get a smart car, this would have to be the one for me. This way, at least I could lead my own parade wherever I went. Instead, I got my medications adjusted to allow me to see well and got a Parkinson's friendly car.

A few months before my diagnosis, I lost my very best friend in the whole world, J. We were kindred spirits, inseparable for over twenty years. Having lost both my grandparents and my best friend all within an eighteen-month period, along with losing my practice and my health, I was not sure I would survive. Yet, it was my friend's words of love and wisdom which resonated with me at my darkest hours, and allowed me to carry on. The last time we saw one another I was a complete mess, having already lost my grandparents and with my grandmother's PD, my new symptoms were weighing heavily on my heart. I was beginning to be concerned about my future as a doctor and so on, but my friend told me, "I don't worry about you because I know that no matter what happens, you will always land on your feet! You are tough as nails," and then suggested the idea of me becoming a writer. After I sold my office, I took my friend's words to heart and each time doubt invaded my mind about my capabilities, the faith my friend always had in me gave me strength.

Now my new friends whom I have met through PPAC, as well as my old friends, all have become irreplaceable; thus proving the old adage: "When God closes one door He always opens another." Therefore, we have to be ready to embrace all that is new and uncertain in our new world with Parkinson's.

Besides having a great friend to stand by us in times of need to share the good and the bad, we also need to be savvy about our financial futures. Most of us are not business gurus and even when we are professional women we might rely on our husbands or significant others to make decisions concerning our futures, like where to invest our money or even if we should invest. More than ever, we have to have basic financial sense when we are faced with a lifelong chronic illness that not only is going to require a lot of planning and large monetary sums to provide for us and also for our dependents when we no longer can provide for them. Second, every women needs to have her own savings bank account independent from any other shared accounts with husband, partner, etc. Taking care of you is as important as taking care of everyone else. This does not have to be a secret, not fostering disharmony in a relationship but rather, peace of mind for you. Financial security not only helps you in a personal crisis but also helps to empower you. When I first stopped working and closed my practice, not only was it devastating having to give up my profession, but I was afraid for the first time in my life of relinquishing independence, particularly financial, and the possibility of being left destitute should my husband leave me since I no longer could provide or support myself. Although I shared joint accounts with my husband, I relied about 90% of the time on my salary for my personal and professional expenses.

Furthermore, I was the one who maintained our home furnishings and maintenance and paid for most of our vacations. The first time I had to go to a bank machine in over a decade, I was a basket case because obviously I did not know any pin numbers. My husband still laughs at this scenario of me calling all in a panic wondering how to withdraw money. Fortunately, I have a great husband who provides and cares for me; nevertheless, it was a wakeup call to what can happen in the blink of an eye. Not only can an illness like PD strike suddenly, but it can cause a shift in the balance of marriage in which everyone is not able to bounce back so easily. Hence, I write about steps to ensure financial security for you and your children, should you lose your spouse.

The best decision I ever made was to maintain my personal account, although I no longer was working. I also chose to invest the money that the sale of my practice brought me. This helped ease my troubled mind tremendously. Now without a source of income, I had to rely on the earnings of my husband, which was a HUGE adjustment for someone who had always been independent and used to earning her own money.

This financial security has allowed me, as it would you, to increase the value of what I do. We as women sometimes tend to undervalue ourselves.[1] Oftentimes we "treat ourselves as a commodity," allowing others to decide our worth, like when a spouse or partner decides to leave the marriage after the wife is diagnosed with PD.[2] You don't have to be the victim, but rather a triumphant heroine even in the face of PD. Take charge of your life by first taking charge of your finances. Consult with a financial adviser, seek the counsel of a lawyer to guide you, so the future, although somewhat uncertain in terms of the disease, does not catch you totally by surprise and you can still be in charge. By the way, Friday is your best bet to get in touch with a financial adviser.[3] Get yourself a copy of the book, Women & Money by Suze Orman. This will be most useful in the fight against a long-term debilitating illness. Not only will your library be enhanced, but you might be amazed at what you could glean from this woman's empowering book, if you are not a businesswoman or have a finance degree. Attend some classes online or at a local institution to get some basic knowledge of finances if you have never had to be on your own. You might even be able to audit these classes. I guarantee it will be the best time spent in investing in your future.

As I stated previously, seek counsel from an estate planner because it is imperative that you have a will, a living revocable trust with an incapacity clause, and an advance directive, which includes a living will, a medical power of attorney, and a durable power of attorney for healthcare.

A will dictates how you want your assets distributed after you pass away; otherwise, the court will decide for you. Not only will the court decide how your assets are distributed, but your survivors (children, etc.) might have to pay some fees. You don't necessarily have to have a lawyer, but I highly recommend having one to write a will. All you have to do is write it, sign it, date it, and two people who watch you sign it must also sign it.[4]

A lot of states have rules as to who can make decisions regarding medical-related issues for those who can no longer make decisions for themselves. However, many states do not have these rules. Therefore, it is essential to have a durable power of attorney. This is for finance purposes, allowing you to appoint someone to act as your representative. This representative is called an "attorney-in-fact." The reason it is called "durable" is because he or she continues to act on your behalf even when you become incapacitated. Therefore, it is important that you specify in great detail the extent to which you want this person to do business on your behalf, such as overseeing investments, paying bills, running businesses for you, etc.[5]

It can cost around $500 to hire a lawyer to write a power of attorney, but not having one can be devastating and much more costly in the end. For those who need to make a petition to a court for guardianship of a loved one because he or she can no longer make decisions, such a petition can cost you upwards of $2,500—and that's assuming the petition is uncontested.[6]

A living trust is a revocable plan that provides for the management of your assets when you die or become disabled.[7]

Advance Directives

1. A living will, also known as a directive, to physicians is extremely important because it allows you to put in writing your own personal wishes about your own medical care if you become incapacitated, unable to communicate, or reach end of life or have end-stage disease.

2. A medical power of attorney, on the other hand, allows you to designate someone to make routine medical decisions on your behalf should you lose the ability to do so on your own. I was my father's medical power of attorney since I knew what was best for him, given his wishes and my medical training. Make sure that you review your will at least every three years. Review beneficiary designation any time there are life changes. Every two to three years, go over estate planning documents to make sure they are all signed and not outdated. Following these simple tips will help give you and your loved ones peace of mind. As the disease progresses, so do expenses. Having a financial plan in place as well as knowing where all the legal documents are kept (keep all documents in an organized binder in a safe deposit box). What the chronically ill person's wishes are ahead of time go a long way to relieving stress in the family, so they can focus on what's important—the care and welfare of the loved one in need!

15

Four Keys to Unlocking Happiness
in the Midst of PD

"When people are serving life is no longer meaningless"
~ John Gardner

We have to stop living life as if it is all about us and realize that what we do matters. Only then will we begin to make peace with ourselves and with an illness that may at times appear as if it might strip us of our dignities but it can NEVER do so unless we allow our SPIRIT to wither. Having been around Parkinson's individuals for nearly three decades, one thing I know for certain is that people with Parkinson's no matter their story or circumstances are as a whole a fighting, determined, generally optimistic group of people. Therefore, I know that when isolation and depression hits, as it invariably will at some point or another especially if you are a woman, it is good to remember that you have it in you to fight back and stand tall and weather the storm. These four tips may be useful to help fight the loneliness and doubts when they invade the mind, and help you keep a positive outlook on things.

Parkinson's is one of those many horrible diseases, I do not wish on anyone. As a practicing neurologist for many years, I have witnessed the devastation of many illnesses. Thinking about all my previous patients always helps me keep my perspective and count my blessings. I have cried at the bedside with parents at the loss of a child due to an incurable brain tumor as often as I have for diagnosing a child with a rare, progressive, relentless, neurological illness that was sure to take the life of their precious child within a few years, sometimes months. I have also felt the pain and agony of a mother bargaining with me and God for extra time to see her children at least graduate high school before she died of ALS. Yes, I may be slow, stiff, in pain, and at times shaky and forgetful, but I can still move and get around; most days I am independent even when it takes me three hours to get dressed. Thanks to my illness, now I have more time to spend with my family, especially my daughter.

So, the **first rule to being happy** is remembering that no matter how hard life seems, or how fast it comes at you sometimes with all its relentless fury, ALWAYS be grateful for the small things. The small things in life truly do matter and do make all the difference. Even when you think no one is watching, a small act of kindness or a smile can make the difference in someone's life. The smile and love of a child can be as powerful or more than the most expensive medicine in the world to a broken heart. The encouraging words of a loved one can serve as the fuel to a burning fire, to give strength to fight and hold on one day longer.

The **second key to happiness** is to continuously challenge oneself to go out of one's comfort zone—even when you feel like people may be staring when you dine out because you are extremely shaky or have trouble getting money out of your wallet to pay or even to sign the credit card bill. It does not matter. Remember, tremors increase with stress so if you learn to meditate or relax before going out, I bet your tremors would decrease. The doctor may also prescribe a mild anti-anxiety medication just for such occasions. Once you are in the presence of friends you will forget about the tremors and will begin to have a good time; however, I am not recommending you become an alcoholic and certainly do not recommend drinking without first discussing with your physician, since some medications may have an adverse effect if taken with alcohol, like Azilect. But this elixir can also help to soothe and calm the nerves and decrease tremors, especially the action tremor type. If hypophonia or decreased voice is a problem for you, then going out to a noisy place would be a perfect setting to practice methods from Lee Silverman Voice Therapy (LSVT).

If you go ahead and take time for yourself, friends, and loved ones, I guarantee you will not regret it and before long you will begin to feel happier and stronger. For instance, with the advancement of PD, I, too, find myself less willing to venture out. Sometimes being a couch potato is just what the doctor ordered—path of least resistance sort of thing. My body appreciates it quite a bit and I don't have to challenge myself in any way, so for a while I seem to be content. However, I recall that is not who I used to be. I was always on the run doing four or five things at once. Contrary to the PD personality theory, which states that people with PD are rigid, controlling, depressive, socially awkward, and morally rigid individuals prior to getting the disease, I was an adventurous soul.[1] I think that the so-called PD personality is a result of the disease and not the other way around; at least this is what I have observed, taking into account my grandmother, my good friend, and my own personality prior to the onset of the disease. Yes, I was a worrier and always measured things before doing them, and like those I mentioned, I have always had my own OCD (obsessive-compulsive disorder) traits. I could not be a doctor otherwise, which by the way, some believe that those of us in the medical field are at higher risk of getting PD.[2] However, these personality traits never stopped me from going parasailing, wanting to go skydiving, or riding in a hot air balloon, which I actually climbed on but was it not meant to be due to a malfunction, or from being the center of attention. Half of the traveling I have done around the world has been on a whim and without much thought as to where exactly it was that I was going or staying, etc. I just went in search of adventure.

My grandmother was quite the adventurous soul herself, and she and my friend with PD were never depressed until they started developing symptoms of PD. However, as the disease has progressed, I noticed a tendency to become less adventurous and more rigid, which I automatically rationalize as fear of being caught in a situation where I cannot help or do for myself. But with a little "mind over matter" thinking, I can almost revert back to my old state of thrill seeking. If I push my body and mind to overcome that initial fear, I find that once I am out and about, I am my old self; it does, however, take some doing at times. However, as far as my moral compass, I don't think that has changed a great deal; spiritual wellbeing was always an important part of my life then, as it is now.

Invariably after resting a while, my mind starts building enough dopamine that I often have to force my body to catch up to my mind. Some days, it is not as easy as it sounds. My husband calls these days "there she goes again, making plans the body can't deliver" days or moments. This poking only makes me want to try harder to prove him wrong. Thus, I extricate myself from my favorite position of "couch potato" to give up the remote control to the TV, forcing myself to get out and exercise to avoid stiff muscles, and if the science proves to be correct, build more/new neurons to avoid cognitive decay or slowing.[3]

Fortunately, I am surrounded by a lot of friends who make sure I stay both physically and mentally active. Furthermore, I volunteer in local and national organizations to ensure I am always being challenged physically and more importantly, mentally, as well as helping others. The biggest challenge that we all face, however, is being able to maintain our functions, abilities, and being able to perform our daily tasks. Until we got PD, we often took simple activities for granted, like putting on our shoes, brushing our teeth, tying our shoes, buttoning our blouses, putting on our underwear or even bathing, much less doing the bed.

Helping others and reaching out to others in need is the **third key to happiness.** I often heard it say if you want to improve yourself, start by helping others. Think of yourselves as salt that mixes with everything. Although apparently insignificant all by itself, it provides zest, it preserves, and it adds flavor to life. When you start helping others you will not only begin to empower them with knowledge, confidence, and love, but you will be adding these things back to yourself—double whatever you give. Random acts of kindness.

The **fourth key to happiness** is patience. I truly believe that you have to be careful what you ask for because you might just get it. Patience was never my strong suit. As a matter of fact, I used to ask God for patience on a daily basis. Guess what?! I got my wish. I got an illness that makes me as slow as molasses, makes my thoughts and gait slow. Everything takes forever. Funny, the thing I no longer ask for is patience. Now, I am just learning to be patient. Since it takes me twice as long to do almost anything, I get many chances a day to practice! Once I was the queen of multitasking, but now performing the simplest activity leaves me utterly exhausted, looking for a quick fix and a nice piece of dark chocolate to boost my dopamine levels. I urge you to learn and practice patience; don't be like me and wait until you have the illness to learn, like the man who use to pride himself on punctuality. One day he overslept and missed his ferry. He was so overcome with fear of being singled out by his boss for being late that when he arrived at the dock the boat was six feet out from the terminal, so he took a huge leap and landed on the boat. He heard from the captain: "Great jump! But if you waited another minute, we would have docked and you could have walked on."[4]

16

Exercise and Parkinson's Disease

"A passive life is not best for the brain."
~ Robert P. Friedland, MD

The year 2014 was one of the coldest in the recent history of the US. It was amazing to witness the power of the winter ice freeze in Niagara Falls almost entirely, because running water is much more difficult to freeze. Similarly, muscles in constant motion are much more difficult to become stiff and experience freezing. We as humans have been created to be active, both in our minds as in our bodies. When we stop moving, this is when we begin to decay.

A story comes to mind of a famous violinist by the name of Paganini. By the age of eleven, he had performed his first concert.[1] Upon his death, after revolutionizing the world forever in the techniques of playing the violin, he willed his violin to Genoa.[2] However, the condition was that the violin would be displayed for all to see but never allowed to be played again by any other artist. With time, this fine and exquisitely made instrument, which had made beautiful music for years, completely disintegrated from years of being unused. It was full of decay and consumed by worms. Yet, other similar violins of the same era were passed down through generations from one gifted musician to another, and continue to this day to enrich the world with their music.[3]

Unlike Paganini's violin, hundred years later these instruments are still intact and play as beautifully as the first day. The difference is not in the wood or the players but in the fact that they are used. Similarly, our bodies with Parkinson's like the violin and other wooden instruments are frail. And like the wooden instruments, as long as they are played they show no wear. Our progressively slower and stiffer bodies, if stimulated, can be maintained for years without decaying. It took years for neurologists to discover that function could be restored after a stroke with the use of physical therapy. I think that similarly with Parkinson's, with exercise and therapy, function can be restored and disease kept from progressing.

First of all, the word exercise is derived from the Latin root "to maintain," "to keep" or "to ward off." Through exercise we are trying to "ward off" disease progression in PD or "maintain" current function by use of various forms of physical activity. One reason we want to exercise is to promote vitamin D production, which has been found in marked deficit across most Parkinson's patients. One-half of all Parkinson's patients have a Vitamin D insufficiency, while a fourth has a clear-cut deficiency.[4] Vitamin D status is categorized as optimal at >30 ng/ml, insufficient at 21-29 ng/ml, and deficient at <20 ng/ml. Vitamin D is not only important in bone stability but also a key component in memory.[5]

Exercise is believed to improve cognition by means of two mechanisms discussed below. In a disease where 40-50% of patients develop memory loss and dementia, I think that it might be a good idea to institute some exercise into our daily routines even if the science has not been completely worked out yet! We know that when mice exercised, the more they ran the higher the correlation to increase in neurons and neuronal activity.[6] We know that with age, certain areas of our brains are more susceptible to deterioration and damage, like the basal ganglia, so perhaps by increasing blood flow and oxygen to these areas and allowing growth factors (proteins that help support the growth in the branches within a neuron) to be released via exercise, we can retard or prevent further deterioration.[7] Exercise is also key in developing and maintaining good bone structure and preventing osteoporosis; hence making us hopefully more resistant to hip fractures and retard loss of bone density. Plus, when we exercise it helps our brain release chemicals that increase our mood, giving us a more positive outlook—this is especially important for us women with PD who according to what we discussed so far have a tendency to get more depressed than the men with PD. Another added bonus of exercising is better sleep as long as exercise occurs first thing in the morning, **not** before bedtime; otherwise, it will have the opposite effect![8]

Just as we do physical exercise, it is equally important to do mental exercises as well. As I mentioned previously, the basal ganglia is a vulnerable area as we age and can begin to falter even worse when disease stricken by Lewy bodies from PD. However, research shows at least in normal or aging basal ganglia, that it can improve its function in relation to coordination and memory when mental exercises are done routinely.[9] Some of the mental exercises that you can do to help you not only feel better but improve your quality of life is mental rehearsing of function or activities—something that most professional sports players, musicians such as piano players, ballet dancers, and even surgeons do on routine basis. When you rehearse in your head a movement like tying your shoes, it goes flawlessly because the body does not get in the way with its clumsiness or stiffness, etc. The more you rehearse in your head and visualize this action being performed, you will soon discover that it becomes second nature by taking it out of the higher-thinking cortex, thus bypassing areas that are damaged by illness and allowing you to still perform tasks—finding a new way of doing things if you will. However, this process takes time and constant repetition. This is especially important for achieving balance and preventing falls. As we know, falls are one of the biggest problems with Parkinson's. Falls due to Parkinson's disease are the second leading cause of spinal cord and brain injury in people over sixty-five.[10]

Exercises such as swimming are top on my list of recommendations. Not only does swimming allow us to stay fit while getting a thorough and complete cardiovascular workout, but more importantly, it helps us individuals living with Parkinson's to combat limb rigidity as well as prevent pain. Another water exercise that I enjoy very much is aerobics in deep water. Getting in the pool serves several purposes: 1) It helps you socialize. 2) You can exercise with minimal effort, particularly if you suffer from back, neck, hip, or other joint pain. The fact that you will not be weight bearing on the joints will make it that much easier for you to exercise. 3) You must be in the deep end, so use a noodle or life vest. If you can tread water for a bit, it helps strengthen core muscles even more. The pressure of the water will help relax stiff muscles.

If you are having balance issues, this is the best place in my opinion to exercise. I was falling a lot at the beginning and once I started this program, the falls stopped. Use a noodle and try to stand on it with both feet; count to ten, then twenty. It will be hard at first. You will fall over, so don't be shocked. The more you do, the better your balance will be. Then I recommend standing on a noodle with one leg at a time for equal amounts. Follow by kneeling on the noodle, first with one knee, then with the other knee for ten counts, then twenty counts each, and then switch to both knees. If you do this at least three times a week you will notice improved results in your balance, decreased falls, and it even decreases dizziness.

Always do these exercises in a supervised environment either in physical therapy with a pool, or in a pool with a lifeguard, and wear a life vest.

Lately there have been reports that walking briskly helps Parkinson's patients improve motor function.

It also confirmed in past study findings of warding off cognitive decline when walking for forty-five-minute sessions of moderate intensity at least three times a week for a minimum of six months. The findings published in *Neurology* were as follows: [11]

- There was a 7% increase in aerobic fitness and gait speed.
- A reduction in tiredness was seen in 11% of the patients.
- Attention/response improved 14% (perhaps because patients were not so tired and actually were feeling better; not as apathetic, along with actual improvement in motor functions).

- Motor function and mood improved 15% (supporting previous studies that exercise is a good antidepressant). When we feel good, we not only have a better outlook on life but also tend to give it 100% more effort than when feeling down or blue in my experience.

Another exercise I would recommend, aside from walking at least thirty to forty-five minutes a week, is tai chi, which you can do sitting or standing for fifteen minutes to an hour at a time, depending on your condition. I recommend trying to find a DVD of tai chi Parkinson's exercises developed by a certified tai chi instructor living with Parkinson's disease. The beauty of tai chi, which often includes sequences of slow movements coordinated with deep breathing along with a deep mental concentration and focus, is that the exercises can be done sitting or standing and in sessions of fifteen minutes to an hour. Even when you start with sitting exercises, you can build up to standing poses. Doing these exercises not only will improve your balance, coordination, muscle strength, and flexibility, as well as improve mood and predisposition, especially if you do them in a social setting. You may obtain your copy by visiting www.parkinsonsexercises.com.

My favorite move is **Painting a Rainbow.**[12] This is for several reasons: 1) because I am always following rainbows—they give me hope when I see one, 2) because rainbows only come after a storm and serve as a reminder that even though I may be in midst of a "Parkinson's" storm at the present, a rainbow bringing joy will soon come out, and 3) I have fond memories of a my dear and sweet friend Martha whom I had both the privilege of knowing as a wonderful human being and as a patient before she went to be with the Lord. Despite having Parkinson's, she never let anything get in her way. Her motto was: "a cup half full not half empty." She was the tai chi instructor for the senior center here in Nacogdoches till the day of her death. She was the one who introduced me and many other participants to this and other poses during one of my Parkinson's symposiums in town to raise PD awareness a few years back.

This is how **Painting a Rainbow** is done.

Overall effect: Imagine turning your head from side to side as you look at something on your outstretched palm, while trying to cover the crown of your head with your other hand.

Raise arms overhead:
- Breathe in
- Raise body
- Draw arms straight up fully extended
- Elbows and wrists slightly bent
- Turn palms facing each other

Turn to left:
- Transfer body weight to right leg
- Turn body to 9:00
- Keep knees slightly bent
- Extend left arm out to left side at shoulder height
- Elbows and wrists slightly bent
- Left palm up
- Turn head to left
- Eyes focus on extended left palm
- Slightly curve waist over towards extended palm
- Curve right arm over head
- Right palm faces down above center of head

Return to center:
- Breathe out
- Transfer weight so weight is equal in both legs
- Draw both arms up fully extended above head
- Elbows and wrists slightly bent
- Palms facing each other
- Turn body from waist to 12:00

Turn to right:
- Transfer body weight to left leg
- Turn body to 3:00
- Keep knees slightly bent
- Extend right arm out to right side at shoulder height
- Elbows and wrists slightly bent
- Right palm up
- Turn head to right
- Eyes focus on extended right palm
- Slightly curve waist over towards extended palm
- Curve left arm over head
- Left palm faces down above center of head

Repeat: *turn to left* thru *turn to right* four times

The next type of exercise that I find beneficial is yoga. I understand not all women can do this. I, too, can only do certain poses, particularly those poses that are beneficial to maintaining and keeping balance. For guidance, I suggest getting the book by Renee Le Verrier. This book is titled: *Yoga for Movement Disorders: Rebuilding Strength, Balance and Flexibility for Parkinson's disease and Dystonia*. It was written by a person living with Parkinson's disease, who is a yoga instructor and has good techniques and advice to improve both physical and emotional balance. I find it easier to do stretching and balance exercises in a pool in the deep end because it helps strengthen my core without physically exerting too much pressure on my already weak back.

Another form of exercise that has been evaluated to a great degree in Parkinson's patients is dancing, especially doing the tango. This form of exercise is the most delightful in my opinion because it is fun, always fresh and engaging. This helps build strength, balance, coordination, and flexibility but also improves mood, hand eye coordination, attention, as well as increases socialization.

Whatever you do, try to combine different activities to challenge your brain and learn new tasks. Don't forget to exercise your brain on a daily basis! One way is to experience and learn new things. One form of exercise that incorporates this is called *Neurobics*, one of my favorites, founded by Dr. Lawrence,[13] which incorporates exercising by way of using all five senses and emotional senses in unexpected ways to avoid your brain becoming complacent and help to make new pathways. Simple things like going to work a different route or shopping at a new grocery store or brushing your teeth with your opposite hand.

Finally, one good way to wake up your brain in the morning while you wait for your meds to kick in, while you are still in bed, slowly begin to move your toes. Stretch, wriggle, and scrunch whichever way feels best for you. Move all your toes up and down several times. This will activate your brain, internal organs, and nerves. Also massage your tummy in circular motion from ribs to pubic area to stimulate your bowels. Doing this first thing each morning will help energize you and become more alert. More importantly, take your steps safely throughout the day to avoid falls.

You might feel old and feeble, but you need a reason to get up out of bed every day. You must always get up and get dressed, even if you are not going anywhere. If you don't, chances are good you will stop caring and apathy will set in. When you feel good about yourself, positive things begin to happen. If you have trouble dressing, use my recommendations from previous chapters. Try to get out of the house. Go out and take a drive. If you can't drive, try running. Some of you, like me, can't run because of doctor's orders but you can still walk even if it's with a walker. But if you do the exercises of tai chi, which you can do sitting, or deep water exercises, before you know it you can be walking with a cane or better yet, unassisted or even flying down on your own two feet! If you have been bedbound, try sitting up. If you can't sit up, wiggle your toes, legs, shoulders, arms, fingers, and sing. Let others know as well as yourself that you are still in the fight and are not ready to give up any time soon. Go ahead, pick your favorite tune, and get dancing! Or you can join a local PD group that incorporates dancing, such as the Spokane PD Dance Group.

Stacie Friend, a mom, caregiver, and woman with YOPD states, "I run because it is a therapy in more ways than one; it helps me with my muscles and mental clarity. Most importantly, I run because I CAN! It is simple . . . just run!"

I also recommend the DVD, *Parkinson's Gettin' Down to Business* by Sherryl Klingelhofer. This DVD is one of several in her collection and is geared towards newly-diagnosed Parkinson's and YOPD. She is also a Tai Chi Moving for Better Balance instructor. About this, she says, "My interest came about when my dad, a retired physical education teacher/coach, developed PD, so together we developed specific exercises for PD in the early 2000s. There was nothing beyond exercise that was helpful for PD, so we set out to make our own. Dad's physician told him that our work was so much more effective than the local PT, so we continued under his watchful eye. I now honor my father by bringing the best information to help make lives with Parkinson's better."

17

Emotional Exhaustion

"Behind every successful woman is a substantial amount of chocolate."
~ Suzy Toronto, www.suzytoronto.com

Sometimes we have not because we ask not. In Parkinson's, like any other chronic illness, learning to prioritize is of the utmost importance especially when dealing with a system that intricately depends on the interactions and input from cerebral cortex and basal ganglia in order to properly regulate pain in the thalamic sensory area of the brain. So, when our brain gets off kilter and dopamine levels start to wane, something else has to change and/or up regulate to compensate for this deficiency. The thalamus does not differentiate between physical and emotional pain. Thus, when we hurt, whether from a broken heart or a broken leg, the brain feels and experiences pain in the same manner.

What often happens, as it did to me, is that we set ourselves up for emotional devastation unknowingly or subconsciously. One moment we are high on dopamine, feeling good and invincible, thinking we are "Wonder Woman," and the next thing, we are crashing, feeling low, and devastated. At times, these feelings can lead us to hopelessness, causing us to be afraid of the future and unable to move forward with our lives. Sometimes, the only trigger is overextending ourselves beyond our physical limitations. We sometimes ignore that soft, quiet, inner voice begging for rest, so we push on. We crave our old life before PD and do not adjust to the changes that a life with Parkinson's demands, and if we are not careful we can become casualties in our own battles.

Thus, it is crucial to remember that Parkinson's is not who we are or what we are, but rather, a part of our life. Other times, we may overextend our limited energy in advocacy just to feel normal . . . but at what cost? Should we ignore our health, neglect our family, or jeopardize our happiness to prove that we can still multitask or that PD is not our boss? The result could be that many of us have become emotionally exhausted, fatigued, weary, and isolated. It is an extremely dangerous place to be in, particularly when Parkinson's already predisposes us to these negative feelings. As women we are more likely to get depressed in general. We are more prone to experience these feelings during pregnancy, menses, menopause, and if we are married. Add to the mix that PD patients can have upwards of 50% of depression at any given time, and we can feel out of control pulled in all directions.[1] Sometimes we unwillingly become victims of the "hurried" syndrome we create for ourselves.

I, too, am guilty of this. After undergoing two major surgeries in a span of six months, instead of resting as I should have been, I kept pushing myself, partially because of family demands and partly because I did not want to appear weak to my family and myself. The consequences were disastrous! I was afraid to say "no" to things that I knew deep down would cause pain or fatigue and would aggravate my illness. I wanted to feel "normal" quickly. I hated the idea of "missing out" on something important because Parkinson's was holding me back. This is crazy, of course. Sure, I missed plenty of nonessential things, which only caused me mental anguish for not being able to partake in those activities at the time, such as not being able to attend the World Parkinson's Congress in Montreal. Yet, the world nor I fell apart because I did not attend. We need to shift our perspectives and instead focus on what we CAN do without harming ourselves and driving a wedge between us and our loved ones, who should come first. Think about the legacy that you would like to leave behind for your family and your children.

After my surgeries, the only thing that happened to me is that I got weaker and extremely fatigued. Subsequently, it took me much longer to recuperate, and I ended up contracting a cardiac virus, which was not surprising given my weakened state. The only natural course that results from fatigue and emotional exhaustion is a decrease in the immune system. Attempting to be strong on my own without asking for help only led to an increased dependence on others with even minor things like dressing due to extreme physical weakness. This entire scenario could have been avoided if I had not forced myself to do more than I could while convalescing. The weariness that ensued from this whole ordeal resulted in greater physical and emotional fatigue as well as severe emotional exhaustion, which is the cycle that leads all of us to poor judgment, cloudy thinking, and poor decision-making.

When we let ourselves become emotionally devastated and depleted as I did, then we are most vulnerable to divorce, suicide, and other harmful, self-deprecating behaviors like gambling, excess shopping, and eating.

I recalled how the wrong combination of medications made me "crazy." Having once before stood at the precipice of the vast abyss staring into the void, I knew I could not travel down this path yet again. Yet, after an entire year of illness, which included a myriad of specialists, doctors' visits, and outpatient procedures, I was truly and utterly spent. I did not know if I had the strength to go on fighting a disease that had taken so much from me already. I wondered out loud if it was all worth it. But the answer, my friend, was and is a resonating YES!!! Nothing in life is final except death. As Marilyn vos Savant best stated, "Being defeated is often a temporary condition. Giving up is what makes it permanent."[2] I opted with the help of my physician who made me confront my mental exhaustion to renew my motto: PRAY, REST and START AGAIN tomorrow!

Here I am in a new year, working on this book. Never would I have thought it possible the way I felt last year, but had I given up I never would have found the strength or the courage. My sweet friend's voice kept resonating in my head: "If you can't practice neurology you must write." So since I sold my practice, I have been trying to learn a new art, sometimes poorly, sometimes enthusiastically, sometimes doubtfully, but always to release a fire which consumes me to encourage and educate, but above all to give a voice and a face to this so-called brain disease of mine. I only wish that through my musings you may also find hope and wisdom for the journey ahead in dealing with your own Parkinson's illness.

Now, I truly understand how many of my former patients, friends, and readers, both young and old, have felt at times of crises. Many, however, have not been so fortunate to make it through to the other side of the valley. I hope that this will give everyone the courage to fight ONE more day! Because I have seen the effects of depression firsthand not just in me but in my friends, patients, as well as in my loved ones, I can honestly tell you that you are not alone in having these feelings. Fortunately, there are ways to combat this problem by actively stopping the negative thoughts. When you dwell on something it becomes ingrained in your brain, akin to walking on a fresh green path. The more you walk over the same trail, the deeper the groove and soon any remnants of green grass will be gone because it has been trampled to death. It will take a very long time for that path to be restored to its former, natural state. However, if you only walk once or even twice in the same path, the trail will soon disappear and will be as pristine as it ever was.

Since PD women appear to be at higher risk, we need to try both physical and mental exercises to ward off negative thoughts and feelings and replace them daily with positive actions such as smiling, singing, dressing up, and simply showing up even if you don't feel like it. Even when you are not in the mood to socialize, don't forget to wear that pretty, feminine color of clothing or a lipstick that brings out your smile. Never under any circumstances when feeling blue or sad should you make any life-changing decisions. Focus on making it through the day. Remember, no storm lasts forever.

Unfortunately, because of society's persistent views on women, particularly in certain cultures, some women may be reluctant to come forward and ask for help when needed for fear of appearing "weak" or being labeled as "crazy," even "hysterical." This frequently happens among the Hispanic female population with issues of mental health. In the case of Hispanic women with PD, this becomes a serious problem, given the fact that as I mentioned before, not only do women with PD have a higher tendency for depression, anxiety, etc., but at least a third of early PD patients present with depression.[3] Now compound this with a possible higher incidence of developing PD among Hispanics here in the US.[4] We are going to be seeing a large portion of PD women walking around this country unhappy, defeated, and sad, leading potentially to a much lower quality of life, which not only will drastically impact the way they view themselves but adversely affect their individual families.

Asking for help takes courage and strength, the opposite of weakness. Deep down each and every one of us women is brave and fierce. I also want to remind everyone that "denial, like depression, certainly has its obvious benefits; however, it's not a healthy place to visit for too long; it can suck you in and keep you."[5] I say that if we can bear children, tend the home, have a career, play doctor, be a wife, mother, and daughter, we can beat depression as well. Letting go and forgetting is actually good for the brain. This is how the brain remains healthy and able to cope with new information and events.[6] But, don't try going it alone; this is not the time to be Super Girl. This is the time to be lifted up and carried by those who care about you the most. It takes a whole family, including the doctor, therapist, and counselor to beat this; the first step has to start with you and your positive thoughts.

Sometimes the best we can do in the midst of the chaos is to stand still and KNOW GOD IS (exists)—Psalm 46:10. Even Jesus, son of God, got tired, worn out, and needed rest. Don't underestimate the power of rest and being still. I often think of it as a necessary step in order to cure or fix what is ailing a patient. Being a doctor, I like to think of this analogy before doing any procedure on my patients. First, I had to make them lie very still to administer the necessary anesthesia/pain medicine in order to carry out what needed to be done, such as mend a bone.

Without rest, we have a tendency to keep going, making us feel increasingly more vulnerable and afraid to stumble, make mistakes, with a tendency to inflate our flaws, thus causing us to not only lose courage but become increasingly isolated and withdrawn.

Similar to a convalescing patient recovering from surgery, an emotionally battered Parkinson's woman also needs all the support and assistance of a team of loved ones, family, and friends to lift and encourage her.

Things you must do when you feel like you are getting bruised, battered, and tired while having difficulty coping with the daily challenges of life and PD:

- Rest.
- Stand still, close to God.
- Engage the help of loved ones (this includes your team of physicians and care providers).
- Increase your dopamine intake during healing and recovery periods. I have found this technique makes a huge difference in expediting the healing process without draining you mentally and emotionally; consult your physician first before making any changes.
- Never, under any circumstances, shut yourself off or isolate yourself.

By following these simple rules, you will find that although the road is arduous, you are able to overcome!

18

Art Therapy: An Alternative Therapy for Treatment of PD

"There are no second acts in American lives."
~ F. Scott Fitzgerald

Fortunately, this statement no longer holds true when dealing with brain diseases of certain varieties or chronically ill individuals, in part thanks to the power of art and the ability God has given our brains and minds to be able to develop great new skills and talents that were never possible prior to our illnesses. Furthermore, thanks to science, in the last thirty years neurology has gone from being a field of mainly diagnosis with little treatment to a treatment-based field, which now offers many patients with chronic illness a chance for a better quality of life.[1] These changes in science and newfound abilities in turn have allowed all of us who have lost something through illness to have a second chance in life, a "second act" if you will, to heal our broken lives and restore our damaged bodies, brains and souls.[2] The idea of second chances and healing through art has never been as crucial in my life as it is now, as non-traditional forms of therapy are beginning to arise as possible new viable treatments for Parkinson's disease, which also holds promise of slowing down progression of same.

As a practicing neurologist, I focused primarily on traditional therapies in an attempt to repair or regain what was ravaged by disease in the nervous system in the form of strokes, dementia, and Parkinson's, to name a few. However, their personal loss was secondary to treating the damage inflicted on their bodies and brains. Yet, I realized this was ineffective therapy because the patient as whole entity with individualized dreams, ambitions, and fears was either not being properly addressed or disregarded entirely. Through my years of practice and in dealing with personal illness as well as that of loved ones, I have learned that if there is no inner healing of a person, there can never be any outer healing, no matter how much a health professional tries. So, slowly I began to help my patients overcome their illness by incorporating nontraditional therapies in additional to the standard treatments of care.

I first became aware of the power of "art therapy" in my grandfather. He was diagnosed with vascular dementia. For many years prior to his illness, he had been an artist. He used to work with whatever media he found at his disposal and that called to him. His favorite medium was wood. He could walk along any path and see a branch of what appeared to be an ordinary piece of an inanimate object that to the untrained eye was only good for kindling a fire. Yet, my grandfather could carve from these discarded pieces the most exquisite sculpture. However, after several strokes had devastated his mind, he no longer could recall the name of my grandmother even though they had been married for sixty-four years. Despite his severe dementia and stoke disabilities, when given a piece of wood or an apricot seed, my grandfather could still carve a most delightful and whimsical turtle or monkey as skillfully as ever. During those moments of active involvement in his craft, my grandfather would suddenly be transformed. For those fleeting moments he would be "normal"—happy and animated in his conversation without a single deficit. For those few moments, I had my grandfather back.

A few years later, I was equally surprised by one of my Parkinson's patients who had a severe debilitating disease with severe tremors, stiffness, and slowness. She required assistance for most of her activities of daily living. One day, this particular patient brought me a beautiful painting she had crafted herself. I assumed she had painted this prior to her illness. However, to my surprise, she had done this in her current condition. Most surprising was the fact that her artistic skills had improved as her disease had advanced. Furthermore, she stated that she felt most content but also "normal" while painting. Other physicians around the world have experienced similar findings.[3-4]

This knowledge continued to percolate deep into my subconscious prior to becoming struck by Parkinson's disease at a young age myself. After the diagnosis, I unwillingly began to experience a certain loss of self as well.

As I continued my journey, trying to make sense of my new predicament, while attempting to use my passion for neurology, in particular, for Parkinson's patients, I discovered a whole host of patients with "de novo artistic" talents. The majority of my patients acquired their artistic talents after diagnosis. These patients' artistic talents ranged from painting, which seems to be the most common form of artistic expression, to sculpting, photography, dancing, and writing poetry. Others used less common methods of expression through music, such as singing, or dancing. Furthermore, on closer inspection I ascertained that these Parkinson's patients were using their newly found or enhanced talents not only to cope with disease, but I found evidence that the art itself was making their disease better. Although there is very limited data at present that indicates that art improves the physical aspects of a chronic illness or a neurodegenerative disability, it appeared that these patients through their art involvement were more active, with less physical impediments. Even more astounding was the appearance of decreased mental and cognitive deficits in these patients than those who were not in "art therapy."

While still practicing, I was vaguely aware of "art therapy" as a means of healing physical impediments left behind from neurological insults like strokes. The art therapy was believed to help strengthen the affected muscles while stimulating the mind.[5] However, I firmly believe it does more than that. In fact, I believe that art therapy promotes the building of interneuronal connections. If one path, i.e., bridge of neurons, is damaged, our brains will force us to find novel ways of expressing ourselves. I have seen aphasic patients who are unable to speak due to a brain insult to the Broca's area, which is the speech area of the brain, be able to speak normally while singing or when speaking in a different language!

Although we have known for years that therapy does not restore dead cells or damaged brain tissue, yet we observe this phenomena as evident in a stroke patient who suffers paralysis after a brain injury and makes a complete recovery after therapy is instituted, while the brain injury remains unchanged.

What is most impressive to me and to those studying this phenomena of acquiring abilities where none existed before seems to be the legacy or aftermath effect of brain pathology. Once the brain has suffered a major insult, through either trauma or loss of brain cells from disease, it appears that offering art therapy can help individuals recover full function, even if it's short-lived as was the case with my grandfather. In more extraordinary cases, the disease or trauma itself can induce spontaneous creativity and artistic abilities after being ravaged by brain disease. The phenomena of developing newly acquired abilities after brain insult is known as "acquired savant syndrome"—where a person with extraordinary talent/skills which they are neither born with or have acquired (i.e., artistic, musical, or mathematical) from a later place or date.[6] This extraordinary brainpower was first described in 1880 after a man by the name of Eadweard Muybridge suffered a severe brain injury, which according to scientists led to the development of his artistic brilliance despite suffering from traumatic brain sequelae and personality changes all of his life. Prior to his photograph, "Horse in Midstride," people often wondered how a horse galloped—if on one foot or all four? These pictures set the stage for his later work in motion picture projection, which never would have occurred had he not suffered a head injury.[7]

More recently in 2003, Bruce Miller,[8] Professor of Neurology at the University of California, San Francisco, discovered that some patients with degenerative brain disease gained incredible artistic abilities as their neurodegenerative disease progressed, particularly those suffering from frontotemporal dementia (FTD) and Parkinson's disease. This confirmed the idea that the brain is not at all static but able to mold, morph, and even surprise us by allowing the so-called victims, i.e., patients, to become victors instead, through *"de novo artistic expression."* Over the last few years, there is mounting evidence, especially with regard to Parkinson's Disease, that suggests that having the disease itself leads to increased creativity and artistic "de novo" phenomena[9, 10] while a select smaller group of PD individuals develop new artistic abilities altogether with the onset of Parkinson's Disease. These new talents and skills have placed these patients in the same category as Eadweard Muybridge and in the elite company of other "acquired savant syndrome" individuals, although not by trauma but by possessing a neurodegenerative disease affecting the brain.

One theory scientists propose to account for this phenomena is the notion that the neurodegenerative disease leaves the unaffected brain alone or rather intact. Therefore, the healthy "unused" brain then is free to STEP UP and compensate for the loss of tissue even though we all use the entire 100% of our brain daily, not 10% as erroneously believed![11] As I said before, there is now growing evidence of de novo artistic expression in patients with Parkinson's and other neurodegenerative diseases like frontotemporal dementia. Even the media is catching on to this idea when they based an episode on a character suffering from FTD as having acquired new artistic abilities as a consequence of his neurodegenerative disease on the popular TV show called *Perception*.[12] Moreover, there is a recurring interplay between brain disease and artistic ability throughout history in the art world. Several famous painters like Van Gogh had neurological disorders.[13] Some claim that Van Gogh had schizophrenia, also a dopaminenergic disease with excess dopamine in the brain.[14] This idea points to the notion of dopamine system being somehow involved in creativity. Other painters like Salvador Dali also suffered from PD while other famous artists like Virginia Woolf, Ernest Hemingway, and Edvard Munch, all great masters in their own right, suffered from bipolar disorder, which also appears to be linked to the dopamine system.[15] We know dopamine is involved because when patients who had undergone DBS were studied, they found them to be less creative, and this was presumably due to the decrease of medication, i.e., dopamine, after surgery.[16]

But, the fact is, like my grandfather who suffered neurological impairment, other great artists were able to cope with the consequences of a devastating chronic illness and persevere in the practice of their art well into the end stages of their illnesses. Not only did they overcome great adversity but the art served as therapy to ward off mental and body decline. The art(s) transformed these great artists from fragmented human beings, who were unable to go on with their lives due to having suffered various forms of trauma, loss, injury, and brain disease, to people of purpose. Oftentimes, these individuals found physical healing through the process of creating art, which in turn led to emotional healing in many instances. Such was the case of renowned artists like Horst Aschermann, Marc Chagall, Georgia O'Keeffe, Willem de Kooning, and Henri Matisse, who continued creating art well into their late years despite suffering from various chronic illnesses![17] Aschermann himself suffered from Parkinson's disease for the last twenty years of his life. Despite his severe tremors, dyskenesias, and rigidity, he was able to produce more than twenty-seven works of art including two large bronze reliefs.[18] Chagall in his nineties became the first living artist to exhibit at the Louvre despite suffering severe depression from his wife's death, the ravages of war and the holocaust.[19] While Georgia O' Keeffe produced beautiful handcrafted clay pots, it was her first time working in this medium despite suffering from severe macular degeneration.[20] Even de Kooning painted well into his nineties. Some of de Kooning's later works include the first painting to be hung in the White House by a living artist despite being afflicted with Alzheimer's dementia. Yet, he was quoted saying, "I paint to live."[21] As the many examples above have shown, art is truly essential for the "spirit" to thrive. This should come as no surprise since the word "spirit" comes from the Latin word "spiritus," meaning breath, soul, courage from the French "esperit," meaning heart and valor.[22] The spirit is that which animates us and gives us our purpose in life despite the obstacles of disease, injury, and loss. It is also that which gives us "courage" to face the unknown, despite the fear and anxiety resulting from loss brought about by chronic disease.

Other famous painters like Gary Markowitz exclaimed, "Painting is one way I connect with myself —my higher self—that spark." His collection of over five hundred works of art produced primarily by mentally ill individuals from all over central Europe[23] underlies the essentialness of "art therapy" in order to bring harmony to any individual who has suffered an emotional, mental, or physical loss. Furthermore, this impressive collection highlights and serves as a reminder that having brain disease or mental illness is not an end to all, but rather a stepping stone for a new beginning for many through de novo artistic expression.

Despite all this new knowledge, we are just barely scratching the surface of the mind and body problems. There should be no doubt about the existence of body and mind working in unison as ancient philosophers believed.

Since I was a little girl, partly because of the influence of my grandfather in my life, I have always enjoyed and been drawn to the arts. I grew up reading famous poets like Neruda. Later it was Walt Whitman but the effect was the same. During my formative years, I spent much time writing poetry and I have always felt at ease surrounded by great works of art by famous artists like Picasso, Dali, Kandinsky, Klimt, van Gogh, Monet, and Renoir whose unique brush strokes along with bright colors and singular shapes appear to launch out at me from the canvas itself. Such was my inspiration that I implemented a lot of these artists' unique colors and styles in designing my own office. I have always felt at home surrounded by color and great works of art. But aside from this, I have never had much in the way of artistic talent or much desire to try artwork on my own.

Somehow after symptoms of PD began, I found myself suddenly having a downpour of poetry which had not occurred in over twenty years, followed by a huge desire to experiment with painting. Granted I am still not an artist but I truly enjoyed the few classes I have taken since my diagnosis, as did my Parkinson's friends from the support group whom I work with. I thought that if I enjoyed art this much and could actually draw something halfway decent despite my severe dystonia and slowness, perhaps they would too. So, I took along my Defeat Parkinson's Support Group here in Nacogdoches, along with Alzheimer's patients who were invited along by my friend Mandy, who was in charge of the area Alzheimer's chapter. No one had trouble completing the task; everyone stayed focused, and each one produced a genuine masterpiece!

Most importantly of all, the social experience was priceless and irreplaceable. Now everyone has their own work to brag about at home to their families as do I. I certainly believe that the artistic side is linked directly to the dopaminergic system. I doubt that it's all medication induced since my artistic side began to flourish prior to starting any treatment when I began construction of my office. It was quite colorful and unique and inspired by my favorite artists. My patients and staff would tease after learning that it was my design behind the colors and decoration and overall flow of the office that I should set up an interior design consulting business—my office needed to be divided into neurology and designing! This interior designing desire has grown stronger since I have been on medication. Hence, I believe that dopamine intake enhances creativity while the disease itself somehow unmasks some innate desire, as some of the Parkinson's people I have gotten to know have affirmed that once disease hit them, suddenly they had an artistic talent they never knew possible, some even without ever having any training. After intake of my dopamine agonists, particularly levodopa, my desire to write and be creative goes up dramatically and declines as that medication wanes in my system. Hence, we can see a Parkinson's patient continue to play the piano flawlessly despite advanced tremors, stiffness, and slowness, even when unable to carry out other activities of daily living.

We are not entirely certain how art therapy helps or increases artistic expression—whether it is through a mechanism of disinhibition that allows us to freely express our most inner desires and thoughts, thus affording us the opportunity to bravely confront our illness without the ups and downs, or because of those nice, positive chemicals released as we do art, or due to the natural changes that occur in our brains as a result of PD. The fact is that all of us benefit from this type of therapy, allowing us to return to our former creative states we once experienced as children. As Dr. Gene Cohen would say, "Art is like chocolate for the brain," and who does not like chocolate?[24] After all, chocolate releases many chemicals similar to dopamine in the brain and if we can get the same effect from art as we do from chocolate, then I see no reason to stop. Now, you can do art anywhere with the new app for art designed to help boost memory as well, called "*GE MIND*" app. You can get it at www.bit.ly/MINDapp.[25]

According to George Land, "We grow up to be uncreative."[26] Children ask a million questions a day as all of you who have children or have been around children know; but as they grow up they ask fewer and fewer questions due to social conditioning in school. We go from asking 120 questions a day at age five to only four questions by age forty. That's a dramatic reduction but perhaps once our brain is free to think out loud again we revert to our naturally creative states.[27] Thus, as anxiety and fear begin to dissipate due to loss of inhibition, the person suffering loss may then begin to truly express themselves once more, allowing true healing to commence. After all, it is said that doing art not only allows one to be more in touch with emotions. Thus, having an emotion attached to a memory will make it long lasting; for instance, we all remember exactly what we were doing on nine eleven because of the deep emotional connection we all have to that date.

Art also helps to develop print awareness (what is written and how it is written), visual spatial awareness, i.e., aware of surroundings, verbal creativity, and visual literacy, which is what helps us see things better and more clearly in terms of their worth.[28] Recently, a study was done on twenty-seven Parkinson's patients who were then compared to the same number of normal individuals, looking at creativity. Scientists discovered that PD individuals had an increase in verbal fluency as well as visual creativity and were frequently outside-of-the-box thinkers.[29]

The key to living with our disability lies in being able to live well with it on a daily basis. Unfortunately, neither art nor medicine offers a CURE for our neurological illness but if we allow art in our lives, it can *transform* us. Ancient shamans as well as medicine men around the world have known this secret for centuries. They, like the many artists I have discussed, discovered that making art offers inner peace and joy by tapping into an individual's creativeness, inspiration, imagination, spirituality, and sacredness by providing hope and fostering spiritual unity, a place of peace, gratification and purpose for one's life.[30] Thus, art can become a refuge for us women with PD to have a chance to use what normally lies dormant to fuel a desire to keep fighting and living with passion.

Creativity and artistic expression can take many forms, such as cooking and becoming a gourmet chef. You can also join art classes, sculpting, photography, writing classes, jewelry making, mastering stained glass, scrapbooking, knitting, crocheting, quilting, embroidering, singing lessons, music or dance classes, anything to unleash your inner creative self. This can bring forth happiness and at the same time give an outlet to release the fear to empower you and make you a stronger woman. Since I have developed PD, I have tried many new things like painting, quilting, jewelry making, and even became a better cook and interior decorator. It was a great honor to participate in the **Parkinson's Quilt Project**, the first global awareness project of its kind in the Parkinson's community through the initiative of PDF's Creativity & Parkinson's Project. My grandmother would have been tickled to death to know her granddaughter was following in her footsteps, since she was a great quilter. Never having quilted before, I was blessed to get instructions from my dear friend Pat, whose mom was a PD patient of mine. The quilt was displayed for the first time at the World Parkinson Congress in September 2010 in Scotland.

Perhaps someday I will learn to play the cello, which has been a desire of mine for many years. Look at the resources in your community for some of these classes; some are free and others are low budget. Look at museums and libraries, as well as Hobby Lobby and Michael's retail store. Usually these places, which sell arts and crafts, also offer classes. Better yet, if you have a talent and there is no class, why not share your gift with others? This way you will have increased social interaction and improved creativity because we all learn from one another; plus, it will boost your mood and increase your cognitive skills. This will enrich your life and bring forth the passion needed to make life worth living. If you think you just are not talented or can't do it because of physical limitations from your PD, let these two very courageous women serve as an inspiration to focus on your second chance at life with PD.

One is Joni Eareckson Tada, who became a quadriplegic after a diving accident and despite all this, she began painting with her mouth and now even sings.[31] The other equally impressive woman who also exemplifies great inner strength, faith, and determination and the power of art to help continue the fight is Peggy Chun.[32, 33] Peggy was diagnosed with a motor neuron disease known as ALS, which robs a person of all abilities while keeping an intact mind. She was a painter prior to the illness. When her disease paralyzed her dominant right hand, she switched to her left to continue painting. Then as the disease advanced and she no longer could use her hands, she began painting with her mouth. Finally, in her last stages of the disease when she was too weak to hold a brush in mouth, she began to paint with her eyes through the use of a computer since these were the only muscles in her body that she could move! She has now passed away to a better life, but her work lives on, as does her courage. Although her art style changed dramatically as her disease progressed, she never gave up and neither should you. Take heart; most of the world's greatest artists, writers, playwrites, and composers have marveled us with their gifts, thanks to their own brand of brain dysfunction/illness, so don't let your brain disease be a hindrance but rather a gift for others to partake in. God makes no mistakes—we are as we are meant to be...so that our destinies are fulfilled, morphing from a caterpillar into a beautiful, blue butterfly!

My daughter often says: "There is no art without heart."

Sacha Whitehead, a woman with YOPD, a mother, and artist, describes her love affair with art: "Art is my everything; it has led my journey through the depths of Parkinson's to the ability to overcome its challenges with the power of the mind. Art takes away some pain, but also empowers me to feel success."

19

Current Treatments: The Good, the Bad, and the Promised Land

"Science has yet to isolate the Godiva Chocolate or Prada gene, but that does not mean your weakness for pricey swag isn't in your DNA."

~ Jeffrey Kluger

We know that Parkinson's is a progressive neurodegenerative disease with no cure to date. However, we have come a long way since 1957 when dopamine was discovered as the main chemical responsible for causing the main symptoms of Parkinson's disease. As an aside, this was one of my favorite molecules to study as an undergraduate; little did I know that someday it would mean much more to me than just a compound on paper. Now, I like to wear my own replica of the dopamine molecule that was given to me by my daughter on my birthday!

Since that time, we have seen an explosion of medical treatments and advances in surgical techniques due largely in part to the "decade of the brain" in which lots of money and focus was shifted to understanding neurological diseases.

Thus, at present we have multiple medications designed to reduce symptoms while allowing increased quality of life of an individual with as few side effects as possible. Particularly because every Parkinson's patient's symptoms are individualized, there may be common threads among certain groups which are more similar than others, due to gender for instance, as I have discussed previously. Although understanding the similarities and differences helps us with treatment plans because we only have one set of medications that are not specific for any one group, adjustments are still required.

Treatment outcome is optimized when combined with other non-medical treatment modalities, such as skilled therapy, physical therapy, occupational therapy, exercise, art therapy, dietary consultation, and spiritual guidance. Of course, trying to sleep well and live in a stress-free environment goes a long way for healthier living as well.

First, we have a number of medications which I will outline below. I am sure most of you are familiar with this group if you are a seasoned Parkinson's patient; otherwise, it will serve as a guide for those who are newly diagnosed.

Second, I will highlight some tips I have learned both as a physician and patient about these medications and treatments, which I hope will be useful to you in managing your life with greater ease.

MEDICATIONS

Class: Levodopa (Gold Standard of medical treatment)

Potential Side Effects: Nausea, dry mouth, dizziness, low blood pressure, dyskinesias, hallucinations, migraines*, high blood pressure, sleepiness, vivid dreams.

Type of Medication	Brand Name
carbidopa/levodopa	Sinemet
carbidopa/levodopa controlled release	Sinemet CR
carbidopa/levodopa orally disintegrating	Parcopa
carbidopa/levodopa/Comtan	Stalevo
benserazide/levodopa	Madopar (Europe)

*I discussed migraines in previous chapter in effects of medications in women. If you experience these, follow up with your physician; higher risk for stroke.

Dreams with all PD classes tend to be very vivid and can be of sexual and violent nature. These dreams can lead to acting out dreams known as REM behavior. If you are experiencing REM behavior, you need to talk to your doctor. I have found dreams to be more prominent and accentuated if you take the medication an hour before bedtime. From my own personal experience, REM occurs more frequently on very busy, active days; also, the theme of dreams usually corresponds to inner feelings of individual at the time.

Stalevo specifically can cause:
- Diarrhea and abdominal pain. If this happens, you need to talk to your physician immediately about discontinuing the medication. This is a rare, idiosyncratic response and it won't go away on its own.

- Melanoma increase, due to Levodopa component. Although being a carrier of LLRK2, which tends to be in women with YOPD, predisposes to other cancers, it may also increase risk of melanoma[1] For all PD patients on dopamine agonists and dopamine replacement, especially those which are carriers of LLRK2 gene, I recommend follow-up with dermatologist routinely, and follow their guidelines. Regarding moles, the best time to have moles evaluated is in the winter and best to do in your birthday suit at least every six months. Know where your moles are located, their size, shape, and color. Have someone look at your back and the back of your neck. If they grow or if they are black or pink—my dad had a pink mole that turned out to be deadly Merkel cell carcinoma! Go to your doctor ASAP. I have had melanomas several times since my PD diagnosis; therefore constant screening, lots of sunscreen, and hyper-vigilance are a must since this is one of the deadliest cancers which can actually be cured if caught early.
- Linked to increase in prostate cancer. 2.4% versus .05%, specific to this medication, but of course not a problem for us women. (2)
- Urine discoloration (orange color). This is normal, no panic but it can stain undergarments easily, so be careful!

Liquid Sinemet Formula (for those patients who have severe fluctuations and have sudden "off" states)

- 1 liter of "coffee grade" water
- Level 1/2 teaspoon of vitamin C crystals (powder form NOT pill form)
- Combination of regular Sinemet 25/100, Sinemet 25/250 and/or Sinemet 10/100 pills, such that the sum of the second numbers (levodopa) equals 1000. Use of generic meds is acceptable.
- Put the Vitamin C in the water, followed by the pills.
- Shake the mixture for about five seconds.
- Let it sit for five to ten minutes.
- Shake it another five seconds.

- There will be pill material suspended in the solution. This is the pill binding. The carbidopa and levodopa have been completely dissolved along with the vitamin C. The pill binding may be filtered out by filtering the solution through WHITE MILLETA brand coffee filters. Usually one liter per filter.
- This solution will yield 1 mg of levodopa per 1 cc or 1 ml of fluid. (Dr. Mya Schiess)

By the way, this is a good gauge of how your digestive system is working. This medicine typically takes about forty-five minutes to one hour, at most one and a half hours to discolor urine. This means it has been metabolized in the system and working, but if it's taking much longer than this, it is a clear indication of an absorption problem which invariably will lead to fluctuation of symptoms and much greater potential for side effects when they finally get metabolized all at once!

Constipation is a HUGE problem with all people with PD and worsened by all medications.

Tips to Improve Constipation Problems
- Eat regular meals, small portions four to five times a day if possible and do not eat dinner later than six p.m. Avoid heavy foods that are hard to digest especially in the evening, like salads or greasy foods.
- Exercise regularly.
- Eat lots of fruit and fiber. It is easy to take tablets.
- Drink plenty of water, at least eight bottles of eight ounces a day, plus juices, such as prune juice.
- Stool softener, e.g., Colace.
- Laxatives as needed, e.g., Miralax, or prescription laxatives, e.g., lactulose.
- Prescription medications to help move bowels, e.g., Amitiza, Linzess. I particularly like Linzess; but it must be taken on an empty stomach early in the morning, then wait at least an hour or two to eat to have maximum effect. Plus, I have found that

it works best if you only take it two to three times a week as opposed to daily. This way you avoid dehydration and cramping due to diarrhea.

- Herbal supplements with spearmint (teas) and peppermint oil. This works great to soothe upset stomach, reflux, and helps gastric motility.

Sleepiness is usually less with this class of drugs than with dopamine agonists, but it is still a common symptom, which can be extremely dangerous. You may feel an irresistible urge to sleep, which may cause you to fall asleep even while eating or driving, and especially if sitting still. There are medications used to counteract this phenomenon, e.g., Provigil, Nuvigil, stimulants etc., but bottom line: if you are not able to function due to severe sleepiness, discuss with your doctor ASAP about alternatives or medication modification.

Nausea is another side effect that is pretty common with most drug classes. Fortunately, most people develop tolerance to medications quickly, lessening this side effect.

Tips to Overcome Nausea*

- Changing meds, e.g., switching to different route of administration, sublingual or transdermal.
- Increasing amount of carbidopa, a.k.a. Lodosyn, to be taken either with every dose of levodopa or as a big single dose all at once in the a.m.
- Taking medication with food, especially high protein, to decrease absorption, i.e., less absorption, less side effects.
- Taking ginger-based products, e.g., capsules.
- Taking domperidone with every dosage of meds. But as I said previously, this can alter a women's cycle and cause irregular menses and high blood pressure as well.
- Taking other antiemetics, like odansetron (Zofran) with every dose or as needed.

- Take proton pump inhibitors i.e., Nexium, with PD meds twice a day.

* Ironically, Sinemet comes from the Latin *sine met*, which means without nausea, and was so named because levodopa without carbidopa caused worse nausea.

Always consult your physician before making changes to your medications and never stop medications without a doctor's approval.

Class: Dopamine Agonists

Potential Side Effects: Nausea, lightheadedness, low blood pressure, hallucinations, sedation, sleep attacks, ICDs (impulse control disorders), withdrawal syndrome, dyskinesias (rare), swelling and weight gain (Neupro).

Type of Medication	Brand Name
apomorphine	Apokyn
bromocriptine	Parlodel
pramipexole	Mirapex
pramipexole dihydrochloride ext. release	Mirapex ER
ropinerole	Requip
ropinerole extended release tablets	Requip XL
rotigotine transdermal patch	Neupro

The biggest issue with **apomorphine (Apokyn),** which is the only injectable given under the skin used in the treatment of "wearing off" episodes, is that the initial treatment has to be done in a supervised setting like a doctor's office because it can result in severe nausea and vomiting, requiring anti-nausea medication. It can also cause sweating, drowsiness, headache, yawning, and runny nose, as well as potential lightheadedness, along with swelling, redness, itchiness, and pain at the site of injection. Apokyn can interact with a number of medications;

therefore, it is important to discuss all medications with your physician before getting the medication. Fortunately, Apokyn now has 24-hour nurse assistance to help guide patients and they will even come out to nursing homes or place of residence if questions arise to eliminate fear of using the medication.[2]

Neupro can cause:

- Hypervigilance and hyperarousal, disrupting one's sleep pattern. When I first started this drug, I was "wired." I felt like I was on a boatload of caffeine with tons of energy, requiring very little sleep if any. Fortunately, this side effect is transitory and wears off in a few days. A 1 mg patch is indicated for RLS but can be a good starting point for those of us who are hypersensitive to medications.

- RLS (restless leg syndrome) as well as leg cramps with sudden cessation or skipping a dose.

- A topical rash that appears to be idiosyncratic. Yet, even in those who initially don't have a rash, sensitivity can develop in the skin especially in the areas of frequent use, and also can later experience some numbing effect in that area. I find that larger doses or patches are more likely to cause this sensitivity, particularly if placed on the upper body. Sometimes after twelve hours, I rotate sites, therefore diminishing sensitivity altogether. But always make sure it sticks on the next location. Otherwise, you will experience severe sweating; this is usually my clue the patch has fallen or tangled up in my clothes somehow.

- Low blood pressure, especially as you increase the dose.

- Sleep attack, which is an irresistible urge to sleep, causing people to suddenly fall asleep at the most inopportune times, even while eating or driving.

- ICDs, or impulse control disorders. These are abnormal behaviors described as "failures to resist or control impulse drive, or temptation to perform an act that is harmful to a single person or multiple groups including self"[3] This impulse control disorder or tendency to lose control can be a huge problem that can lead to problems in both personal and interpersonal relationships if not recognized and addressed properly.

It is also important to note that there are gender differences in presentation when dealing with ICDs. Too much dopamine can cause excessive behaviors that were once in check, like pounding or fascination with meaningless objects and activities, overeating, e.g., overindulgence, binge eating, increase in thrill-seeking behaviors like engaging in activities with multiple sex partners (hypersexuality) or increased interest in pornography, gambling, impulse shopping, reckless driving, and hoarding. These aberrant behaviors are more commonly seen with Mirapex (pramipexole) and Requip (ropinerole) and to a lesser degree with Neupro (rigotine).

All behaviors occur more often in women than men except for the sexual and gambling problems![4] I personally believe this is an extension of our own emotional need for control of our surroundings. I have found that these behaviors are a reflection of what is already in us but are heightened and magnified during stressful situations and are more likely to occur as a result of dopamine withdrawal during times of physical, emotional, and mental stress when we are pushing our brain's dopamine to the limit.

For instance, I love to shop and do so whenever I can but a lot of times when I go I have such a discriminate taste that I often don't buy anything. Lately, since I fatigue easily, shopping and browsing do not pair up well. Needless to say, shopping is becoming less frequent for me. However, I have noted that during these last few months, which have been particularly stressful for me, I not only have gotten an intense desire to shop but have started spending like crazy. This had become my comfort zone in dealing with a dying father. Once it hit me that I was using shopping to make me feel better and cope, I increased my dopamine intake and found a more constructive way of replenishing my physical and mental exhaustion through meditation and art therapy. The shopping urge stopped. The same applies to periods of increased sweet craving that is always related to dopamine being used up faster than I am taking, like when I spent days at the hospital with Dad. I would forget to take my medications on time and I would notice an increased need for chocolate and it would then dawn on me I had skipped a dose or several doses. Interestingly, there seems to be a greater occurrence of these types of behaviors in Europe, followed by the US, then Canada, for reasons unknown other than perhaps purely speculative on my part due to time of drug introduction into market, outside US first?[5]

New proposed treatment for some of these behaviors is a medicine called Naltrexone.[6]

Class: COMT Inhibitors

Potential Side Effects: Abdominal pain, back pain, nausea, constipation, diarrhea, blood in urine.

Type of Medication	Brand Name
entacopone	Comtan
tolcapone	Tasmar

People on **Tasmar** must have liver function blood tests routinely. In addition to enhancing the effects of levodopa, COMT inhibitors may enhance side effects of levodopa including dyskinesias and other side effects described in the section on levodopa. Main thing in this category is urine discoloration and diarrhea. If you experience diarrhea, I recommend discontinuing the medication. This is not a side effect that will go away. Urine discoloration can stain undergarments. HELPFUL TIP: One way to remove these stains is by using Pink ZOTE soap which can be bought at most stores where they sell Hispanic products.

Class: MAO Inhibitors

Potential Side Effects: Dizziness, agitation, nausea, rhinitis, headache, back pain, stomatitis, dyspepsia

Type of Medication	Brand Name
selegiline or deprenyl	Eldepryl

| selegiline HCl orally disintegrating tablet | Zelapar |
| rasagiline * | Azilect |

*Additional potential side effects of Rasagiline are: postural hypotension, hypersensitivity to sunlight, and indigestion.

Insomnia is most common with **selegiline**. I recommend taking it no later than one p.m.

The main thing with this drug class is that sexual problems can arise in women, as I described in previous sections, especially with Azilect. Azilect can also cause some urine retention; this can worsen urinary infections if already prone to having this problem.

Also, we have to be careful with dietary restrictions. Foods high in tyramine, like aged cheeses e.g., blue, cheddar, Swiss, and stilton; red wines; fermented soy products like soy sauce, miso, tempeh, and tofu; sausages or cured meats, e.g., salami, mortadella, beef jerky, and smoked or pickled herring; sauerkraut; and fava beans that are eaten excessively and in large quantities especially with Azilect could result in hypertensive crisis with severe increased systolic blood pressure (top number) more than 180mmHg or higher and diastolic (bottom number) less than 120 mmHg, causing severe headache, nausea, vomiting, anxiety, sweating, rapid heart rate, and shortness of breath. If this occurs, seek immediate medical attention.

Always discuss with your physician before making any changes to your medications or diet.

One of the best things about Azilect that I have discovered as a physician and patient and confirmed by some of my colleagues in the field is the untapped potential for use to treat pain in PD. My pain, which was excruciating when I was first diagnosed with Parkinson's, ceased completely after beginning treatment with Azilect. Although Azilect appears to have some very quirky side effects in relation to the female body, I still think it is a great drug and although it did not meet criteria for protecting the brain from deteriorating, many of us neurologists feel that time may prove otherwise.

Class: Anticholinergics

Potential Side Effects: blurred vision, dry mouth, constiptaiton, urinary retention.

Type of Medication	Brand Name
benztropine	Cogentin
trihexylphenidyl	Artane
procyclydine compounds	Kemadrin/Arpicolin (not available in US)

This class once was the "*go-to*" class of meds, since it is the OLDEST class, but now due to newer treatments, these medications are not as widely used especially in the elderly population because they tend to cause a lot of memory problems and "fogginess." Thus, this group of medications is not good for those with PD dementia or the elderly. Yet, as a whole, they are great for tremors and for dystonia due to "wearing off" or "peak-dose effect."

Class: Other

Potential Side Effects: Dry mouth, constipation, diarrhea, dizziness, nausea.

Type of Medication	Brand Name
amantadine *	Symmetrel
rivastigmine tartrate **	Exelon liquid, pill, or patch

* Additional side effects of Symmetrel include urinary retention, ankle swelling, and a mottled skin rash (livido reticularis, which are purplish stripes usually in legs) typically in the legs that goes away with stopping the medication; memory loss. It can cause depression and mood instability as well.

**Additional side effects of Exelon include weakness, drowsiness,

difficulty sleeping, loss of appetite, headache, weight loss, upset stomach, and increased sweating.

Amantadine is commonly employed for dyskinesias and aside from treating tremors, it is a great medication for chronic fatigue.

Exelon is the only FDA approved drug for treatment of PD dementia to date. The biggest limiting factor to treatment with Exelon is the GI side effects, which are fortunately dramatically lessened with the approval of the patch. However, the patch, like any other topical medicine, can cause some soreness and redness at the site and sometimes can cause a severe rash. I have found that cleaning the site with betadine prior to putting on the patch dramatically lessens the likelihood of developing a rash.

SURGICAL TREATMENTS

DBS (deep brain stimulation) is by far the greatest advance in the treatment of Parkinson's disease we have to date. DBS is a device of "implanted electrodes" deep in the brain known as the basal ganglia that provides a continuous, small, electrical current to these parts of the brain in an attempt to "jam" or "obstruct" signaling between malfunctioning, either too much or too little activity in the brain structure.[7] No one really knows the precise mechanism of action at the microscopic level. This not only offers patients improved quality of life due to improvement of symptoms but also "buys" them time if you will until a cure is found. Although extremely effective when done properly, and known to be state-of-the-art therapy, it is neither a cure for PD nor does it replace or repair abnormal brain cells!

Unlike its predecessors—thalamotomy, and pallidotomy—which were surgical interventions targeting the same affected lesions as DBS, producing similar results with one big difference—lesions in DBS are not permanent! Pallidotomy and thalamotomy surgeries are still in practice but more common outside of the US and used especially for those that have a difficult time traveling to a center to have adjustments done.

DBS, which is made by Medtronics, has been around since 1986 and the FDA approved it first for essential tremors in 1997, then for Parkinson's in 2002, and for dystonia in 2003.[8] At the beginning, the indications were much narrower; with time they have been expanding as are the patients who receive this treatment. This used to be a treatment reserved as a last resort but now from years of practice, we neurologists and movement disorder specialists have understood that preservation of quality of life is of utmost importance rather than rescue a patient from severe disability. But, in order to do this, we as patients and caretakers need to start discussion long before disability sets in.

There are still three criteria for DBS for Parkinson's to ensure best outcome:

1. Patient must have idiopathic Parkinson's.
2. Motor symptoms, which must be responsive to Levodopa, are at some point either inadequately or inconsistently controlled with patient's current regimen, which should be at optimal levels.
3. Patient is troubled by their motor symptoms and/or their medication effects. It is very important as well to have a good support system and be able to travel to get programming.

Remember, early education is the key to a successful outcome. DBS is not a cure but can significantly alter a patient's and, therefore, a caregiver's quality of life! DBS is the only treatment to date known to stop tremors 100%. Other benefits include reduction in bradykinesia, motor fluctuations, dyskinesias, rigidity, and improved tolerability to medications. However, I must caution that most people, especially with bilateral implantation, will experience increased speech problems, drooling, gait difficulties, swallowing, cognitive problems, depression, and instability. So, if you already have these problems, you need to outweigh the risk because it is almost certain these will intensify and worsen.

As we discussed previously, PD patients have a higher than usual rate of depression especially in women with PD. Good news, however, is that we do not have a higher-than-general population rate of suicide; it is rather on par or below. But, one class of Parkinson's patients has stood out in recent studies to be at higher risk for suicide. This is among those who had undergone DBS, especially if they either had a history of depression or were single.

The above information is one more reason for you to discuss with your physician your entire medical and psychiatric history in detail as well as your social status prior to proceeding with this type of treatment. (9-13)

PROMISING NEW TREATMENTS

- Another treatment in the horizon is **Focused Ultrasound**, a treatment employing ultrasound waves to create targeted zones of therapeutic thermal injury, which theoretically would target the same areas of the brain and improve symptoms the same way as surgeries without having to undergo surgery. This would be perfect for those of us who are high-risk candidates for surgery due to multiple medical problems, and also for those who are not able to travel to get frequent programming.[14] So far, studies have shown significant improvement in tremors, reducing them by more 50%.

- A new medication making headlines, but not yet approved in the US is **safinamide**, an MAO-B inhibitor. This is a new drug which extends the "on" time of Levodopa in both moderate and advanced disease of PD. Dyskinesias also were reported to improve with this drug. Subsequently, an application for FDA approval has been submitted as of May, 2014 to get the drug approved as an add-on to levodopa therapy as well as for early PD.[15]

- Another drug that has been long-awaited and talked about, **intranasally applied L-dopa,** continues to hold great promise to bypass the GI tract, which is known to be the cause of not only many of the side effects, like nausea, caused by levodopa that makes it hard for patients to take but is also the leading cause of variability of drug performance due to gut absorption.[16]
- **Duodopa pump**, which has been available in Europe and Canada was recently approved here in the States in early 2015. This is comprised of a gel that is infused continuously via the intestines through a pump. My personal belief is that its use will be limited to treatment of patients who have advanced disease and severe motor fluctuations, like dyskinesias, when current available treatment options for PD have not provided adequate responses. Marketed by AbbVie as Duodopa.[17]
- However, the biggest news in the field of Parkinson's is the recently FDA approved treatment for Parkinson's psychosis. This drug called **Nuplazid (pimavanserin)** is an agonist of the serotonin 5-HT2A receptor, believed to play an active role in psychosis. This is in sharp contrast to the traditional approach of treating psychosis with dopamine antagonist, which was known for the most part to worsen Parkinson's symptoms. This could prove extremely beneficial since women with PD have a lot of negative symptoms, including psychosis. As a whole, about 40% of people with PD are said to suffer with PD psychosis, which includes visual hallucinations and delusions. These delusions are oftentimes the infidelity type. PD psychosis usually is associated with PD dementia, in my experience. This treatment is developed by Acadia Pharmaceuticals.[18]
- Another drug currently holding promise is **Dynacirc CR (isradipine)**, a calcium channel blocker medication used for treatment of blood pressure. This is being studied under the STEADY-PD III trial (Safety, Tolerability, and Efficacy Assessment of Dynacirc CR for PD). It is being evaluated for potential disease-modifying qualities, i.e., stop progression of PD.[19] This

is the most exciting study in my mind going on because for the first time a study is focusing on recruitment of minorities and looking at gender differences, plus it is a study propelled forward by PD patient initiative in conjunction with the various major Parkinson's organizations. Now open enrollment @ UT HOUSTON. Principal investigator is Dr. Mya Schiess.

- The promised land of **gene therapy** is another treatment on the horizon. This is a method by which a piece of nucleic acid is introduced or inserted into a brain cell of interest using a "vector," better known as a carrier or transportation system like a virus, that has been changed so it won't cause disease in those who will receive the therapy. This gene therapy has been deemed both a cure and beneficial for the brain type of agent in the treatment of Parkinson's over the last decade. However, for all its hype, it has fallen short of its promises and expectations, leaving many people disappointed both in the scientific as well as in the Parkinson's community. But we have not seen the end of this treatment modality. Gene therapy still remains a promise and a virtual mess that needs to be untangled in my opinion. Within its realm, we may still unlock the potential of slowing down the progression of the disease and find new and improved ways of enhancing the effects of Levodopa, which includes better tolerability and fewer side effects. This could hold the key to individualize medicine, particularly when dealing with gender differences. So, don't dismiss this yet.

- Will there be **a vaccine** for PD? This is based on the premise that PD could be caused by an infectious protein, a.k.a., a "prion-like" disease.[20, 21] A vaccine is currently in phase 1 of trials, evaluating safety. Many in the field of Parkinson's hope that if this proves to be safe to go into phase 3, it will be a disease-modifying or preventive treatment. Only time will tell.

In the end, aside from taking a full medicine regimen on a timely daily basis, is trying to find the right mix of medications along with finding a suitable lifestyle that accommodates your specific needs and ever-changing Parkinson's symptomatology that is influenced by the weather (especially cold), stress, lack of sleep, and other medical issues as much as possible.

RESTORATIVE BENEFITS OF PERSONAL TIME

- Learn to listen to your body. Rest if you must. Increase medicines in times of stress, either physical like undergoing surgery or emotional during a bad breakup or stressful project. Once the stressful situation is over, there is no need to continue with higher doses of medications, but always remember to discuss with your physician first before making any alterations to your medical regimen. This strategy is what I have found to work for me and my patients.
- Through many years of practice, I have witnessed firsthand as well as from a patient standpoint, the restoring power of a five-minute break. Think of it as a mini-vacation or a time-out to pamper you. This simple act, which can be done anywhere, anytime, and costs nothing, can go a long way to replenishing your dopamine levels, reducing your stress levels, as well as decreasing fatigue. There is also biblical truth to this method, for those of us who are more spiritually oriented. *"Be still and know that I am God"* Psalm 46:10. Taking a time-out not only helps restore your dopamine, hence improving your physical wellbeing, but it also helps us focus more clearly on what really matters by listening to our inner voices. I find that healing always comes from within first, and must start there to be long lasting. When you take your five-minute break, think of it as finding that place deep within you, where no matter what storms are raging outside, everything lies peaceful and still within, like an angry ocean—at the surface the waves are constantly changing in all directions to the whim of the winds but several feet below the surface the waters are always calm. Don't allow yourself to be

influenced by everything and everyone around you; stay in your own solitude of peace. Here you will be rejuvenated because it takes energy to go against the winds to fight against our chronic illness. Learn to embrace it and make the best of it by building your inner diva.

- Of course, every diva should get a massage at least once a week as another nontraditional form of therapy, which I have found to be extremely beneficial at keeping symptoms at bay, particularly those of pain and stiffness. Although at present there are no studies to support this type of therapy, anecdotal evidence is mounting, supporting the benefit in Parkinson's patients. Many of my patients and friends with PD have turned to this as their illness has progressed, finding it extremely therapeutic. For me it has been one way to control my pain symptoms without having to escalate my medication dosages. Aside from decreasing my need for pain medications and my rigidity, getting a massage helps keep my immune system elevated while helping me decrease my stress levels. There are very many different types of massages. I prefer the deep tissue massage and so do most of my friends with PD. A Swedish massage does the same techniques as deep tissue without being as forceful and kneading as deep into the muscles. It is the most common type here in the US and for most would be the most beneficial not only to help relax the muscles and decrease pain subsequently. But, according to the *Journal of Alternative and Complementary Medicine* and *The American Massage Therapy Association*, the Swedish massage helps to increase immune system boosting cells, known as lymphocytes, to help the body fight harmful substances and decrease stress hormones. Do not get a massage if you have or had CANCER! Since not yet approved as a standard treatment modality, most insurance plans do not cover. A few do cover massages for health reasons with a prescription by your physician; therefore, check with your insurance to see if this is one of the benefits they cover.

20

Nutrition Matters in PD

"In this {my} house the entire food pyramid is made of chocolate."
~ Suzy Toronto, www.suzytoronto.com

Looking good makes us feel good and vice versa. When we have an illness like Parkinson's, which directly affects our outward appearance, "looking good" becomes an important factor in how we relate to ourselves and others. But it's no easy task. Besides the physical changes of the disease itself, we must also battle the depression, which can lead to overindulging and adding a few extra pounds, and our medications themselves, as they can caused fluid retention and increased weight. Therefore, it is imperative we learn to have a healthy relationship with food.

We know that men and women metabolize food differently. Many of you may share the frustrating experience of going on a diet, depriving yourself of all those "tasty" foods, and losing a few pounds, if you are lucky . . . while your spouse minimally reduces his diet and loses twenty pounds in a heartbeat. This experience can be devastating to our egos and self-image. It is even more disheartening when both you and your spouse are on the same medication; he loses another fifteen pounds, while you are acting like a ravenous beast eating everything under the sun. How is this fair, I wonder? It is not. And no one ever said it would be. So we must play with the cards we are dealt. No reason to pout . . . *okay, maybe just a little.*

How we metabolize food changes as we age and our estrogen levels drop or as we become menopausal. During menopause, we may become more sluggish. Therefore, we must learn to adjust our diets to fit our individual situations.

Our family traditions and culture also play a role in how and what we eat. As I was reminded not long ago while I was giving a talk to Hispanic patients with Parkinson's, one individual told me, "Doctors just want to treat us all the same way. But we are not the same." An important point!

For instance, a Hispanic person such as myself may need to cut back on fatty, greasy foods, substitute flour tortillas with corn tortillas, and try to do more grilling, baking, and broiling to be able to digest food easier. In my culture, as well as in many Mediterranean countries, we typically don't eat dinner till after eight p.m. This time schedule for eating perhaps needs to be scaled back a few hours, if we are to improve our digestive systems. It is particularly difficult to digest a meal, even if it is not fried, if consumed at ten p.m., especially when there is already a tendency for slowness of GI motility for patients with Parkinson's. This "late eating" is typically the number one culprit for my GI problems most every time I visit my family. Other cultures may be big on cheese, other dairy products, or pastas, which also slow down motility, while others may consume large quantities of cured meats, like salami, which may interfere with certain medications and even predispose us or cause us to develop adverse reactions to our medications. We have to become savvy as to what we can and cannot eat, taking into account our cultural predispositions. Thus, dietary recommendations for PD should fall under customized medical care.

I am sure each and every one of you has heard that protein is bad for PD patients, either from your doctors or other patients in support groups. Well, this is not necessarily the case. Heavy protein intake can be a useful tool, for instance, in those of us who suffer from severe nausea or other side effects due to the medication. Remember, in Parkinson's as in life, it's never all or nothing. We must learn balance in all aspects of our lives starting with our eating habits. In general, protein intake becomes more of an issue in patients who have motor fluctuations; otherwise, it does not make that much of a difference in the absorption and release of the medication.

Having said the above, what is the optimal nutrition strategy for women with PD? Unfortunately, there is no one right answer. Each of us will be on different medication regimens, have different food preferences, and experience a variety of gastrointestinal problems related to our own unique Parkinson's presentation. For instance, one woman may have more constipation, while another may have a slower motility and greater trouble emptying her stomach. Someone else may have severe swallowing difficulty or severe reflux, and yet another individual, like me, may have a combination of all of the above. Therefore, each one of those patients requires a unique approach to her symptoms, including diet changes, which include how, when, and what we consume, along with medication changes. It is important to note that dietary changes alone may not resolve all of our GI problems. Hence, seeking treatment from a specialist in this area (gastroenterologist) in conjunction with a dietician and neurologist will provide maximum benefit.

As I have treated many patients with Parkinson's over the years, and now being a patient myself, I have learned that:

1. One GI symptom, such as reflux, does not preclude you from having another one, like constipation. Sometimes H. pylori can be present, which aggravates GI symptoms, also making absorption of medications such as levodopa more difficult.[1]
2. Initial nausea with medications typically subsides within a few weeks. If it persists, then you need to be evaluated for other causes of nausea.

More than what you eat, a routine in meal intake is imperative and trumps all other dietary changes. It is important to maintain a schedule, not skip meals, and not eat late. It is best to eat five to six small meals a day and your latest meal no later than six. And this still may be too late in the day for a lot of us who have severe slowing of our guts. This is the hardest thing to do; trust me, I know! It requires a lot of discipline to be able to keep a routine or maintain a meal schedule, especially when you are traveling, caring for others, working, feeling unwell, etc.

Along with being able to maintain a schedule for eating, it is important to keep well hydrated, particularly during the winter and times of stress. Most of us forget that water is a nutrient! Water helps to dissolve the vitamins and minerals our body needs.[2] Remember, blood is also mostly water, so dissolving these compounds makes it easier for the body to distribute the nutrients to where they are needed. Water also helps lubricate joints, mouth, eyes, flush kidneys, and remove waste; the more water, the less likely you will be to get obstructed.

The best diet that I have found to help me as a PD patient as well as other PD patients is one that is followed by patients with irritable bowel disease or inflammatory disease (IBS), like ulcerative colitis (UC) and Crohn's disease (CD). This makes perfect sense since some of the Parkinson's variants carry a gene believed to be related to other inflammatory diseases, like those I just mentioned, thus supporting one of the theories of Parkinson's—that the illness is triggered by an autoimmune process.[3] I firmly believe there is something to this theory, particularly since I am an LLRK2 carrier and had a diagnosis of IBS in my younger years. Hence, I am well familiar with the diet, which goes something like this:

A typical diet for a patient with UC will be:

- **Breakfast:** an egg, one slice of bacon, a piece of toast, and eight-ounce glass of fruit juice. No milk.
- **Snack:** a cup of fruit, or one-half of a peanut butter sandwich.
- **Lunch:** any meat product with vegetables, juice, and more fruit or Jell-O.
- **Snack:** crackers with one slice of cheese, or graham crackers.
- **Dinner:** portion of meat, vegetables, beans, and a piece of pie.

The main goal in this diet is frequent small meals full of vegetables, proteins, and fruits, with no salads, minimal dairy products (maybe once or twice a week at most) and very little in the way of breads and pastas (maybe once a week).

This type of diet is easy to digest, has lots of nutrition, is balanced, and does not leave you feeling deprived. Because most of the foods are not processed, they are readily and easily absorbed and easy to pass through the colon, decreasing the bulk; plus, all the fruit, water, juices, grains, and vegetables improve motility significantly. Discuss with your GI doctors and movement disorder specialists to see if this type of diet would benefit you, as it has me, and ask if you need a referral to a dietician to help stick to the diet plan with greater ease.

Dietary Recommendations
- Limit alcohol intake.
- Avoid alcohol, which contains high indigestible carbohydrates, like beer.
- Clear spirits such as vodka and gin with water/soda flavored with fresh, suitable fruit; moderation is preferable.
- Drink plenty of water.
- Eat in moderation; small, frequent meals.
- Chew your food well.
- Limit processed foods.
- Fresh fruit, vegetables, grain, nuts, whole meats, and fish are best. Most meals should contain these.

However, nutrition is not just what we put into our body; it is our relationship with food. This latter part is what really matters because once we have an understanding of how we react to food and why, we will then be able to truly enjoy food, and life, to the fullest. After all, not only is food important for personal preservation, it is also a way of bringing people together in many cultures, including my own.

The mere thought of chocolate causes our brains to start producing dopamine. Consumption of chocolate has been shown to release quantities of endogenous dopamine, according to research at the Georgia

Health Science University. This fact has prompted many scientists to find treatment for Parkinson's disease using chocolate.[4]

Because of the powerful intrinsic release of dopamine and calming effects of chocolate, a dark piece of chocolate now and again, at least once a week especially after a massage, will not only help your Parkinson's symptoms but will allow you to feel like a QUEEN! According to an author, artist, and women's advocate Suzy Toronto, "Behind every successful woman there is a substantial amount of chocolate." Second, chocolate, especially dark, is full of flavonoids, which are beneficial to the brain.[5] Third, consumption of chocolate has been shown to release yet another chemical known as serotonin, which is also believed to be involved in patients with Parkinson's. Dysfunction in the release of this chemical is what leads to depression, especially in women. Serotonin is the compound or chemical used to treat depression. This, again, may be a physiologic reason why we women tend to reach for chocolate as comfort food more than men, since it provides a natural antidepressant affect. Particularly, I noticed in myself, my grandmother, and other women with PD, an increase in cravings for "chocolatey" treats during times of stress, both emotional and physical, as well as when medications have worn off. This may be an indication for us all to be more vigilant of our medication intake schedules. If we are reaching for chocolate to increase the endogenous/intrinsic production of dopamine as a supplement to our drug therapy, this could be a sign of poorly controlled PD or fluctuations in our non-motor system, just like dyskinesias are a manifestation of fluctuations in the motor system. My observation of increased chocolate cravings in me, my grandmother, and friends with PD has also been noted by other PD experts. This was confirmed by the survey of 498 PD patients and their partners.[6] The speculated cause of increased chocolate cravings is believed to be due to the anti-Parkinsonian effects of the medication.

Dopamine has also been shown to boost brainpower by increasing blood flow to areas of the brain involved in memory and thinking. Some think it is due to the caffeine-like effect of chocolate.

This effect is so powerful, in fact, that a study of sixty older individuals conducted at Brigham and Women's Hospital in Boston revealed a 30% boost in memory and thinking abilities among those with previously impaired blood flow after consuming hot cocoa twice a day for a month. [7] I, too, find that a cup of hot cocoa (especially dark) is very effective in helping me relax, focus, and sleep better at night.

Drink your favorite chocolate elixir, once hailed as "the elixir of the gods" by the Mayans, in your favorite cup, one that inspires you. Five hundred years ago, this ancient civilization could appreciate the benefits of this raw substance known as the cacao bean. Even my iPhone cover shares my love for the bean: *"Neurologist powered by chocolate!"*

I have a collection of cups—fancy ones with gold trim and others with affirmations that I use to empower me while I relax with my hot, dark cocoa drink! My favorite one, of course, was given to me by my daughter: *"Designated DIVA!"*

Some of you may have too many tremors to drink out of an ordinary cup, especially with hot contents, but you can still enjoy a good cup of dark hot cocoa by using some of these ideas:

- Get fancy, colorful, hard plastic cups and fill only halfway to avoid spilling,
- Use those one-pound weights on your wrist, as I described previously, to dampen your tremors.
- Invest in a cup with a rotating handle designed for people with tremors.
- Invest in cup called a Kangaroo cup designed by an 11-year old girl for her grandfather who has PD—you can get one of these cool looking cups and help raise money for Parkinson's as well at www.imagiroo.com/buy.

To wrap it up, our brain loves chocolate for five excellent reasons:

1. It releases dopamine, making you happy, and helping you learn.

2. It releases serotonin, boosting your mood.
3. It releases caffeine, improving memory, focus, and concentration.
4. It releases tryptophan, helping to reduce stress in your life—helping to reach that inner diva. The smell of chocolate alone decreases brain waves triggering relaxation.[9]
5. It releases flavonols, which create effects similar to those of mild painkillers, like aspirin, so that you can accomplish what needs to be done—basically everything when it comes to caring for your family and loved ones.

Note: Overall, dark chocolate is healthier because it has more cacao; it also contains antioxidants that help decrease blood pressure by widening arteries to improve blood flow; eating dark chocolate decreases risk of heart disease by one-third.[8]

Although chocolate is great **brain food**—and as I and others have noted, because it grows on trees, it could count as a fruit—it can still wreak havoc with your waistline. Consume in moderation and discuss with your physician if you have other medical issues, such as diabetes, where chocolate consumption may not be advisable.[10, 11]

CHOCOLATE RECIPES

There Should Never be Truffle in Your Heart and Mind
as Long as You Have a Friend with Chocolates! [12]

Mexican Hot Chocolate

I like to make my hot cocoa like my grandmother use to make it,
preferably in a clay pot.

- Place 4 cups of milk and add a whole bar of chocolate "Abuelita"
  and 2 sticks of cinnamon, sugar to taste.
- Place all ingredients except the sugar in a clay pot. A regular pot
  will also do, but cooking in clay cookware can give food an added
  unique flavor.
- Place over medium heat and let it begin to simmer, stirring
  constantly with a wooden grinder until all chocolate dissolves
  and milk begins to boil.
- Add sugar to taste.
- For darker chocolate, add 1 ½ bars.

Grandma's Chocolate Cake

Ingredients:

1 cup sugar
2 cups all-purpose flour
4 teaspoons baking powder
1 cup milk
2 sticks of butter
4 eggs
4 teaspoons of Hershey's cocoa powder
1 teaspoon pure vanilla extract

Directions:

1. Preheat oven to 350. Use baking spray with flour on two 8-inch round cake pans.
2. In a medium bowl, beat the butter and sugar. Once smooth, fold in eggs and mix. Slowly add the flour while continuing to mix. Add the baking powder, milk, cocoa, and vanilla. Mix well until all combined. Beat at medium speed until smooth.
3. Divide the batter evenly between the prepared pans and bake for 30-35 minutes, or until a cake tester comes out clean. Cool cakes for about 25 minutes, then invert onto a rack to finish cooling.
4. Set one cake rightside up on a serving platter. Using a spatula, spread strawberry marmalade (preserves) evenly over cake. Top with the second cake and frost the top and sides with chocolate frosting. Add pecans liberally.

Chocolate Frosting:

Ingredients:

Jar of strawberry preserves (marmalade)
2 cups of halved pecans
2 cups powdered sugar
4 teaspoons Hershey's cocoa
1/3 cup milk
3/4 cup milk
3/4 stick of butter
2 teaspoons vanilla extract

Directions:

1. Soften butter, then combine sugar and mix well.
2. Slowly add milk (don't make it too runny).
3. Add cocoa and vanilla. Mix until smooth using medium speed. (May add extra cocoa to make it darker).

Grandma's Mole

Ingredients:

1 whole chicken in parts
1 jar mole Dona Maria
1 bar of chocolate "Abuelita"
1 teaspoon of sugar
Salt/pepper to taste
2 sticks of celery
1 clove of garlic
5 black peppercorns
1/2 onion chopped
3 bay leaves

Directions:

1. Place 5 cups of water in large pot. Add chicken, garlic, onion, celery, peppercorn, bay leaves, salt/pepper. Cook over medium heat for 45 minutes.
2. Sift bay leaves, celery, onion, garlic, and peppercorn.
3. Take out a cup of chicken broth and place in a medium bowl. Then combine mole and mix until smooth. Then, add back to pot with rest of chicken and broth.
4. Add bar of chocolate and continue to cook over medium heat, stirring frequently until chocolate dissolves completely.
5. Add sugar.
6. Add more salt and pepper if needed.
7. Turn heat to low and simmer for another 15 minutes.
8. Serve hot. Garnish with either banana slices or pomegranate seeds.

Fun with the Girls White Chocolatini

Ingredients:
> 2 oz. (60 ml) of Godiva white chocolate liquor
> 1 oz. (30 ml) of Smirnoff vanilla vodka
> Ice
> Dark chocolate shavings

Directions:
1. Frost the glass by putting the glass in freezer for several hours. Frost the vodka as well.
2. Add some ice to shaker.
3. Add the cold vanilla vodka to shaker.
4. Add the Godiva white chocolate to shaker.
5. Shake ingredients, to mix and chill completely, until the metal of the shaker turns frosted.
6. Serve in chilled glass and garnish with chocolate shavings.

Victoria's Ultimate Chocolate Smoothie

> 2 Hagen dazs bars (with or without almonds)
> 1-1/2 cups milk
> 2 cups ice
> 2 tablespoons Quick chocolate mix

Combine all ingredients in a blend and mix on high. For a more liquid consistency, add more milk.

Mom's Pecan & Chocolate Chip Oatmeal Cookies

Ingredients:

2 sticks butter, softened

1 cup brown sugar

1/2 cup granulated sugar

2 eggs

1-1/2 tsp vanilla extract

1-1/2 cup all-purpose flour

1 teaspoon cinnamon powder

1 teaspoon baking soda

1/2 teaspoon salt

1 cup sweet chocolate chips

1 cup pecans cut in small pieces

3 cups of Quaker Oats, quick and uncooked

Directions:

1. Heat oven to 350.
2. Beat together butter and sugar until soft.
3. Add eggs and vanilla, beat well.
4. Add flour, baking soda, salt, and cinnamon. Mix thoroughly.
5. Slowly stir in oats, chocolate chips, and pecans. Mix (best with spatula).
6. Make tablespoonsful of the mixture into round balls and place on ungreased cookie sheet.
7. Bake 10-12 minutes or until golden brown. Let cool for a minute or two.

21

Caregiving in Parkinson's

"If you find it in your heart to care for
somebody else, you will have succeeded."
~ Maya Angelou

I believe this is an extremely important chapter since at the beginning of this book I discussed:

1. Parkinson's incidence increases with age.
2. In the aging population the ratio of men to women is disproportionately in favor of women.
3. Women are also the ones with fewer economical and financial resources, particularly as they reach retirement and the elder years.
4. Women make up the largest number of caregivers even when they themselves are ill.

According to a National Family Caregivers Association (NFCA) member survey, the profile of caregivers is deeply skewed towards the female gender.[1] Women make up 82% of all caregivers, mostly in their homes—80%.[2] Women are the primary providers for their children, their spouses, and their parents—19%, 48%, and 24% respectively.[3] I, too, experienced firsthand what it was like to be a care provider—even as it tested the limits of my patience and skills because I was part of that number who are ill and still called upon to be the caregiver to someone.

During the writing of this book, I took care of my beloved father, who was battling a rare type of skin cancer—Merkel cell, which is even more aggressive and has a higher mortality rate than melanoma. He recently passed. Being the eldest, as well as the physician in the family, naturally most of the medical decisions fell on me. In the midst of trying to balance my life with all of its demands, I was always on pins and needles waiting for the phone call to tell me my father had gone to be with the Lord, particularly when he'd reached the terminal stage and was in Hospice care. Meanwhile, I had a teenager who required my full attention and a husband who was also dealing with the responsibilities of being a caregiver to his own elderly parents, who live even farther away than mine, while trying to continue caring for me and my illness. As you might imagine, the stress level in my house could not have been any higher.

The first challenge of caring for someone other than your spouse is living several hours away even when the caregiver is healthy. Imagine having a chronic illness yourself, like I do, having to deal with Parkinson's and traveling multiple times a week to visit a loved one and lend a hand to the primary carepartner living with the person who is ill. The thought alone of traveling back and forth can wear a person out. During the summer of 2014, while my dad was hospitalized for nearly three weeks, I was at his bedside day and night. Although I took my medications routinely, I was not eating, sleeping, or moving much; sitting in the same, hard, hospital chair waiting to talk to all the doctors took a toll on my health as well. Sometimes the emotional stress can be compounded by a feeling of under-appreciation by the person for whom you are providing care. The exhaustion can begin to cloud your thinking and emotions begin to run rampant, akin to the emotional exhaustion I spoke of before. Due to poor judgment, feelings of resentment can begin to build if we are not careful. It's no surprise that in a poll conducted in 2009 of 1,500 caregivers, 17% described their physical state as well as their emotional state as poor compared to only 13% of the general population.[4] I have experienced emotional anguish firsthand, particularly in dealing with my dad's illness. When we start getting oversensitive, it is a sign of being overly fatigued as a caregiver. This characteristic indicates a burnout. If you begin experiencing this, I suggest taking a timeout to reenergize; if symptoms do not improve, it may be time to get professional help. Remember that you will be no good to those who depend on you if you fall apart. I personally had to withdraw for a couple of weeks to reboot. Taking a timeout lets you appreciate small things, such as enjoying a drive for the first time in months.

A big majority of caregivers are ill themselves, especially when we are dealing with older patients. So, the sheer stress of having to tend to someone else's needs when you, the caregiver, is sick can aggravate and even worsen the symptoms of the diseases of both you the caregiver as well as that of your loved one or person you are tending to. No wonder so many caregivers suffer from depression and hopelessness, especially when they have been at it for five years or longer. Unfortunately, according to NFCA, this makes up over 60% of the caregiver population.[5]

The second challenge is caring for someone around the clock; even when you have help, the mere intrusions of having well-intentioned "strangers" there to assist you in your home day in and day out can wear on you. When my grandmother was living with us, I was running a full solo neurology practice, building a new office, and raising a three-year-old child while trying to care for my grandmother, who had end-stage Parkinson's disease. At that time, I did not have Parkinson's, but I had undergone back surgery. Thus, it was difficult for me to move my grandma due to her illness because of potential flair-ups of my back condition. Yet, being constantly surrounded by "sick," needy people was beginning to wear on me, and I could begin to recognize the same "blank," "lifeless," "emotionally" drained look in the faces and eyes of the primary caregivers of my Parkinson's patients and other family members of patients with other chronic neurodegenerative illnesses like Alzheimer's, etc.

When caregiving seems too much to bear for one single person or family, this is the time to consider these next few points in deciding whether to continue care at home or place loved one in a facility such as a nursing home:

- Family limitations (children at home who require attention, time constraints, money issues).
- A caregiver's physical and emotional state may already be weakened or completely depleted because of personal illness since a big number of caregivers are also patients and/or have children to tend to.
- A patient's illness or condition may require level of care out of the expertise of caregiver.
- Financial constraints (caregiver must maintain outside employment to provide for loved one's care).
- Layout of home may be unsuitable. Patient may need special equipment, for instance, that may not fit in the home.

When it is time to weigh these types of decisions and emotions, a support group along with the assistance of a social worker comes in handy.

For me, sometimes the first order of business when decompressing is getting our home in order. It is amazing how a house falls apart in one's absence or when your full attention is on caring for someone else. For example, something as simple as getting food back in the house is of utmost importance for my family, because I didn't have time to go grocery shopping. The end result is always extreme happiness, especially for my daughter.

Next on my agenda is to catch up with one of my closest friends, Lori, who is a total diva and fashionista like I am. We make it a point to get together at least once a week. The purpose is to talk about other things besides PD or other medical issues, although sometimes the subject cannot be avoided. No matter what the topic of the day is— whether it is the latest novel by one of our favorite authors, upcoming movies we must see, or one of our latest shoe acquisitions—talking with

Lori always makes me smile. She knows I have a weakness for shoes but can't wear just anything because of my PD, so she serves as my scout, looking for cute, colorful, comfortable, and easy-to-wear shoes.

The crucial thing is having great friends to help carry the load of our illnesses, friends who share our burdens, whether these are from the standpoint of caregiver, patient, or both. Meeting to socialize is a wonderfully healthy thing. Lori and I often chat over a cup of coffee, although admittedly mine is more sugar and cream than coffee. According to some studies, frequent consumption of caffeine increases reaction time and improves gait in people with PD.[6]

Finding time to socialize with your girlfriends is not always easy because sometimes all you want to do is stay in bed and hide under the covers, especially when you are sleep deprived, feeling sad, overstressed, financially burdened, and emotionally fatigued. Sleep is important so don't neglect this in order to socialize; your support group will be there after you get some rest. However, don't seclude yourself for too long.

The third challenge is being a caregiver in the "sandwich generation," which means caring for parents and children at the same time. The stress can increase exponentially if the "meat" of the sandwich, if you will, is already frail and sick too. My advice to you is to *get up, get dressed, and make an effort* to participate in whatever activities or functions your family is having, especially those of your children. A positive attitude and demeanor will always generate a positive action, not only in you but in those around you.

Besides your cheerleader group which loves and supports you unconditionally sometimes, I find attending a women's Bible study or a women's support group can provide a lot of spiritual comfort. It always seems to me that, no matter what circumstances I am going through, the Bible study is exactly what I need to lift me up. During a recent Bible study, as I was dealing with my illness, my father's imminent death, in-laws moving to my hometown, and my teenage daughter's itinerary, I felt pulled in all directions. Appropriately, the study was the book of Thessalonians—a book full of hope with teachings on how to cope with disappointments in life, relationships, and how to deal with life's heartaches without losing the fire and love within. I highly recommend reading this study by Beth Moore on the book of Thessalonians, called *Children of the Day*. This can be purchased through LifeWay.com, as well as other book retailers.

Having been a primary caregiver of my grandmother and now an active provider of care in my father's illness, I have learned not only the importance of loving deeply because time is short, but I have also learned about the needs of a caregiver.

Caregivers want most help with or information about:

- How to keep their loved ones safe at home. The majority take care of loved ones at home, 37%
- Managing own stress to avoid going down slippery slope of depression themselves, 34%
- Easy activities to do with their loved ones for whom they care, 34%
- Finding time for themselves, 32%[7]

The stress of being a primary provider can be even more devastating when there is an impact on financial resources, such as not being able to work outside of the home, usually caused by the fact of having a major responsibility such as being a caregiver. This is the recurrent scenario across the country in those taking care of PD patients.

Of further concern is the fact that at least 40% to 50% of all PD patients develop dementia, the consequences of which can be devastating for both the caregiver and patients alike. The increased burden of caring for someone with dementia inevitably spills over into the community and society as a whole. This is particularly true when women are the caregivers because at some point the needs of the patient are no longer able to be met by the caregiver herself with consistency, especially if she has a chronic illness like Parkinson's disease as well. In this situation, the impact on society may be doubled since both may need care in some type of long-term facility such as a nursing home, assisted-living facility or other similar facilities.

According to the NPF, the average number of tasks required for a caregiver to perform doubles in the mid stages of PD disease and triples by the late stages.[8] These rapidly escalating demands on behalf of the patient drastically increase a caregiver's stress, leading to severe depression predisposing the caregiver to an ever-increasing risk of suicide, particularly if mentally and emotionally exhausted due to physical illness. This type of emotional fatigue could push a carepartner to desperation. Hence, I call for an increasing demand for all communities to develop strong Parkinson's support groups along with use of social workers for all PD families. I further highlight that all of us who are caregivers to exercise much-needed "alone time" to avoid negative thoughts and resentment against a loved one. Remember, your health comes first! Think about what you are told before a plane takes off when flying on an aircraft, "*In case of an emergency put on your oxygen first and your life vests, then assist those who need help!*" You cannot be a lifeline to someone else if you are sinking as well. Typically, when the carepartner's quality of life declines, so does the quality of life of the patient. Learn to take time for you to avoid burnout.

As a caregiver to my grandmother and dad, I experienced moments of frustration as many of you certainly have. The reason for this mental anguish is caused by our own internal struggles of assuming what is best for those we are tending to rather than what they may think is best for themselves in the situation they are in.

So, exactly how do we decide when to step in and when to watch from the sidelines, cautiously holding our breaths? This question is an extremely complicated one—deciding when to override their needs and desires for safety's sake. For example, my dad was very frail, getting extremely weak, and had fallen thrice but still insisted on using a walker instead of a wheelchair, which made me cringe.

It is important not to fall into a trap as a caregiver of assuming what the person with chronic illness or PD needs or wants. It would behoove us to ask our partners or loved ones what their wishes are. An honest and frequent dialogue can go a long way in maintaining the personal dignity of the care recipient, your loved one, as well as that of the carepartner who will not come across as a tyrant but rather a truly caring individual.

As a carepartner, there are six important strategies to master to make living and caring for a Parkinson's patient or anyone with a chronic illness.

- **Learn to compromise**—avoid disputes and old issues from getting in the way.

  During chronic illness, especially as a loved one reaches end of life and end-stage disease, this is the time to stick together in order to help him/her feel like he/she still has some independence. So, instead of forcing the wheelchair, in the case of my dad, I explained my concern of him falling again. In a situation of a demented or mentally incompetent patient, sometimes you have to make a decision that your loved one will still want to fight, as in the case of my grandmother, who was bed-bound in the end stages of her disease and highly confused—she would accuse me of holding her hostage. First, you must not take this personally—remember, they are ill. Second, this is when knowing their wishes ahead of time helps. Therefore, as I mentioned earlier in this book, it is imperative to set out durable medical power of attorney and wills ahead of time before cognitive changes set in. I also suggest the support of a social worker with whom you have built a rapport to help navigate these challenging times.

- **Reiterate your concerns in a compassionate manner.** In the case of my father, I explained to him that his bones were frail and weak, and any small, apparently insignificant injury, even a simple bump from sliding off the bed, could lead to a fracture. However, if he chose to not use the wheelchair, then we had to have another safety plan in place. So, he was instructed to call someone first, prior to getting up either from bed or sitting, to alert us of his intentions of wanting to be mobile. He then was to sit at the side of the bed for a few minutes, rather than jumping up and moving forward. These recommendations were meant to safeguard him from getting orthostatic, dizzy, and falling.

- **Learn to coordinate.** Some of us are better at this than others. If you are good at delegating and seeing the big picture, this is your calling. Nothing is more important than having a game plan! For instance, since I am good at this . . .

While my mom tended to the daily needs of my dad, I could step back, analyze what other things needed to be done, and assist my mother in dealing with them, such as insurance, all kinds of paperwork, and scheduling. Were all documents in place? Were wills done? Will there be someone overseeing the funeral arrangements, if dealing with end-stage disease and terminal disease? Are other legal documents in order?

As we know when we are dealing with the task of caring for someone 24/7, we can become so overwhelmed we sometimes can't see the forest for the trees. This is especially the case when death is imminent; our judgment can become clouded, and we may become paralyzed with grief! Be the one who initiates conversation and steers it in a positive direction to get things done that need taken care of. But don't feel like you have to go it alone. Use the help of resources available in your community and lean on your friends during these difficult times.

- **Learn to facilitate.** Emotions tend to run rampant when dealing with a chronically ill loved one. It is hard to step outside your situation and see things objectively. This is when a friend, pastor, social worker, healthcare professional; or in my case, a relative who does not live there all the time, comes in handy. They will/can provide valuable insight into the situation, give impartial advice to diffuse a stressful situation by offering prayer, and even referring you to counseling services, support groups, other resources online, and to other community organizations that may be able to assist with specific needs, i.e., help find a sitter.

- **Learn to listen.** This is the most difficult task of all! Some of us hear but don't really LISTEN. Listening takes special skills, understanding, and putting oneself in the other person's shoes. When we are in a stressful situation, we all desperately need to be heard so everyone talks, but no one LISTENS!

  Oftentimes, no words need to be uttered at all to have truly listened and made the person you are caring for feel special, unburdened, understood, and loved. Sit together listening to music, watching a favorite program, coloring together, reading poetry, looking at old pictures of family . . . These are but a few examples of what you can do.

  The caregiver also needs attention and to be heard; therefore, if you are a person outside of the PD household, ask the caregiver to tell you their story. This simple act can allow the caregiver an outlet to relieve stress, to open the door of communication leading to opportunities to offer assistance if it is desired.

- **Last but not least, learn to socialize.** Again, if you are a leader or a take-charge kind of person or event planner, this would be right up your alley. After all, we are social beings, most of us, even the shyest of us; we thrive when we are bonding with others either individually or as a group. Therefore, it is important to plan social outlets to get the patients out of their stressful situations from time to time to avoid depression, loneliness, feelings of helplessness, and spiritual exhaustion, which might lead to suicidal ideation, but also to remind them they are individuals who have unique talents and gifts. These activities are just as important and sometimes even more significant for the carepartners.

  Caregivers also need to steer clear of negative and self-deprecating feelings which may be brewing within after years of self-sacrificing as a carepartner. The social activities can be done together or separately; it is best if done separately from time to time. Organize activities for the patient which include family and/or friends—perhaps they can entertain your loved one while you get some needed rest. Don't forget that PD women even in our late stages still like to look pretty and enjoy outings. You may have cars customized to make loading and unloading of patient easier, especially if wheelchair-bound. A doctor's prescription can save you some tax dollars in customizing your vehicle or adding wheelchair lifts in back of vehicle. Make sure to continue to allow the Parkinson's woman to get her hair and nails done. There are many services that can come to the house if the patient is housebound, or maybe you and your family can do this as a special treat. When my grandmother was living and since she was bedbound we were limited as to what we could do. Yet, one of the favorite things she enjoyed and I enjoyed doing for her was doing her nails and hair and putting makeup on her. This made her feel less ill and more alive. Sometimes, even my three-year-old at the time would get in on it. My grandmother did not mind playing makeup with her; rather she relished the time together even if her nails were a mess and she had blue eye shadow all over her face.

Do include some personal socializing on your own away from the patient, such as hanging out with friends to talk or go shopping, a movie or even a nice mani-pedi. Put your imagination to work. Even if it means going out for an unexpected treat, like an "ice cream" run. I had a Parkinson's patient whose thrill was just this. In my dad's case, his joy was fishing, even if it was just in a bucket, I'd suspect.

Take a timeout for your family's sake especially if you, too, are a patient. Use those girlfriends, which I said every woman should have, to lift your spirit, build you up when you are down, and help shoulder the burden when it gets to be too much to bear alone.

No matter what may come, keep your mind alert, your dreams alive, and your body moving! As beloved author, poet, and woman activist Maya Angelou wrote, "*Plant a kiss on the cheek (of your loved one) . . . so they can continue to count the action as natural and expected.*" [9]

Taking into account all of the above advice, to be a successful caregiver is to be accepting. The sooner we learn that this "too shall pass," the sooner we can move forward with what and who is really important.

As a dear friend, Marjie Hughes, long-term caregiver to her Parkinson's mother, told me once, "Take time for you. As the caregiver, it is very important that you take care of yourself physically and mentally. You will be no help to the one you love and are caring for if you don't. Do not allow yourself to feel guilty if you take some time for yourself. You don't know how long they will need your care."

Cathy White, long-term caregiver, devoted wife, and friend to one of my sweetest and oldest Parkinson's patients, has said this about being a caregiver: "Caregiving can be the most frustrating and most rewarding thing you will ever do. Be sure to make time for yourself whenever possible. Your loved one may at one time blame you for their situation as their condition progresses and will take their frustration out on you, but just hang in there. At some point Hospice may be necessary—accept their help; and remember that you have done the best to care for your loved ones every step of the way."

22

Wrap-up

"You are braver than you believe, stronger than you seem, smarter than you think."
~ Christopher Robbins

Given all of the experiences and knowledge discussed in this book, we know that Parkinson's disease today is no longer the same disease of our grandparents. What I knew as a Parkinson's specialist about PD is no longer the entire story. For instance, PD does not affect the dopamine chemical only. Plus, the disease is no longer confined to the basal ganglia, as it once was believed. Now it looks like PD may be a very complex systemic disease starting elsewhere outside the basal ganglia in regions of the brainstem and/or the olfactory nerve simultaneously[1] causing the pre-motor symptoms or early clinical symptoms like sleep disorders, loss of smell, depression, and visual changes. Moreover, we are learning that women and men with PD not only may look different at presentation but also may behave differently throughout the disease. Some still think that YOPD has a lower rate of occurrence; anecdotally from my own experience this appears to be changing. Although PD is mostly sporadic in nature and only 10% of the time is it caused by genetic abnormalities, or familial, those who carry the LRRK2 gene appear to be of Ashkenazi Jewish decent.[2] But overall, women with PD are credited with having a slower progression of the disease, especially in young onset, reaching stage 3 years later than male counterparts of similar disease onset.[3] At the same time, we are requiring less medication overall. Remember, we are more prone to side effects at doses given to men; perhaps overmedication at the onset of diagnosis is one of the reasons why women with PD have more dyskinesias?

Clearly, we PD women have been plagued with more of what experts term "negative" or non-motor symptoms, such as apathy, depression, pain, etc. This terminology may be a misnomer given to women perhaps by those who have been looking at Parkinson's disease in women as a glass half empty instead of half full. Thus, the solution to treating women with PD may be as simple as a shift in our focus as neuroscientists and Parkinson's specialists. This may require a revamping in our thinking to better understand who it is we are first in the context of gender, followed by our ethnic origins and cultures. When we begin to focus on these three areas, we may begin to uncover traits which may be useful to diagnose and treat all Parkinson's patients. Patients in general are more apt to respond to treatment modalities once their unique characteristics are taken into account. In establishing a plan of treatment for women with Parkinson's, for instance, we should take into account things like hormonal status (i.e., menstruating or postmenopausal) and support/family systems. I submit that by focusing on the differences instead of the similarities among PD patients especially with regard to gender, we might be more likely to find a cure for various subtypes, if not all PD patients. As was the case not long ago for a certain type of breast cancer: once scientists began to focus on the outliers and differences in the presentations of the breast cancer, they were able to identify a familial gene now known as the "BRCA gene" which proved to be responsible in some women for an increase in breast cancer risk.[4] Once this mutation was known, specific recommendations were able to be made based on this gene type, along with modifications to the treatment of breast cancer in all patients, especially for those who carry this gene.

One such modification for PD women might include less levodopa for body weight in women, or treatment with immunosuppressants or anti-inflammatories for certain disease types like LRRK2; since those carriers of LRRK2 appear to have other diseases which are inflammatory or autoimmune in nature (e.g. bowel disease in the form of ulcerative colitis and Crohn's).[5]

Since specific strategies have not been implemented to treat PD according to subtype or gender, at present all PD patients' treatments to date are guided by symptoms.

Although the role of hormone interplay in Parkinson's continues to be murky, it is clear from reviewing the literature, that it DOES play a role in women's PD since PD symptoms worsen with menses and vice versa.[6] How big and until what age is not clearly understood. As long as we continue to downplay the role that hormones exert in the behavior of women with Parkinson's—not just estrogen but other hormones such as oxytocin, which causes us women to react differently to stress compared to men—we are always going to be missing a piece of the puzzle when it comes to treatment of women with PD. As the study conducted by Liu et al of 119,166 postmenopausal women suggests, no hormonal factors have been universally associated with an increased risk in Parkinson's disease across all domains.[7] Yet, female hormones continue to be implicated in Parkinson's development in one manner or another as we observe those who undergo an early hysterectomy develop an increased risk of developing PD. Plus, women who received postmenopausal hormone therapy have been noted to have a reduced associated risk of PD. At least on the surface, as it is in brain and heart disease, estrogen appears beneficial for the protection of the brain's activity.

Prominent movement disorder specialist Dr. Plotkin agrees that "women do present differently in some respects and may be a sign of an 'entire new novel entity' different than your typical Parkinson's disease."[8] However, as he and others have confirmed, we don't have enough data at this point to support such allegations. Hence, we are in the process of trying to increase data collection by whatever means necessary to better understand this disease process in women and in particular, young women.

With the advent of increasing numbers of young women developing Parkinson's disease and women as a whole presenting and responding differently to standard treatments, we are poised to begin redefining our roles as physicians, caretakers/carepartners, family, spouses, and other ancillary health professionals. How will this new knowledge impact the care and treatment of women with Parkinson's? Since Parkinson's disease affects not only the patient but has ramifications that extend far and wide into the fabric of the community in which that individual lives, we have to be prepared to find a team of "cheerleaders," if you will, to help guide and support us through the ups and downs of life from spiritual counselors to dance instructors and everything else in between. After all, it takes a village to care for a chronically ill patient like me and you. But we don't have to sit idly by waiting for others to make a difference; the power to inspire the next generation of neurologists, who will be taking care of Parkinson's patients like us and working for a cure, lies within you and me. By becoming our own advocates—after all no one knows you like you know you! Not being in control of oneself and feeling blue or depressed is the number one reason why so many women with PD have left the workforce. Sadly, these women with PD also tended to be in the lower socioeconomic group—meaning poor resources and support most likely—exhibited a higher mental stress, depression, and anxiety since their first visit.[12] You alone have the power to change this cycle; before becoming research advocates, volunteers it is important to take care of your own needs. If volunteering in a study like Steady PD III or any other study where you will receive close follow-up and attention will boost your spirit and allow you to feel like you are contributing, then by all means do so. The main goal is to maintain quality of life in all of us women with PD. This includes job retention for as long as possible. Continuing to be productive members of society by staying in the workforce once we are diagnosed with Parkinson's is a heavy burden physically and emotionally for all people with PD, especially for women. We know that work helps to enhance our quality of life by making us feel useful and wanted; however, it has also been noted that motor symptoms actually affect PD individuals a lot less in the ability to continue to work and do the job well, compared to those with non-motor symptoms like depression, anxiety, and pain.[10]

This is where we PD women may seem to be at a disadvantage initially being misdiagnosed, misunderstood, and not included in studies. Also due to a heavier leaning of negative and non-motor symptoms making job retention a lot more difficult for women. Thus our own quality of life can begin to disintegrate from the onset of disease if we don't actively pursue our own happiness and wellbeing by means of alternative therapies such as art, exercise, and meditation along with eating a proper diet with some chocolate of course, not forgetting that style plays a big role not only in society but in our lives individually. Once you are determined to be the master of your own destiny, you will be a force to be reckoned with. Now you will be poised to change the world, make your voice heard. When our voices are heard, it no longer will take five or more visits to be diagnosed. No longer will you settle for symptoms being ignored. Everything you are feeling is real and needs to be addressed by the right specialist.

Learn to have balance in your life.

Yes, there is life after Parkinson's, as you and I begin to "live la levodopa" to the fullest while advocating PD for ourselves and others, maintaining our homes, careers, friendships, marriages, and raising children, learning not to sweat the small stuff.

In order to make the most out of living with Parkinson's and being happy, I have learned to remind myself on a daily basis, if necessary, to prioritize *myself*—and you should do the same. If you are like me as most moms and wives, our needs always come last, especially when you have been in the healthcare profession as I have where your job is to take care of everyone else first. One thing you must never forget: **You are still you, despite PD.** This means that your goals, dreams, and aspirations should not cease because of a chronic illness; rather, they should morph to incorporate the disease and become something greater with a higher purpose. If you were a painter, keep painting; if you were a writer, keep writing . . . yes, it may take longer or may take on a different theme or style, but it is still part of who you are. The Parkinson's is only a part of your life, like the color of your hair or your eyes; it does not define your beliefs, talents, capabilities, or who you are as a person. As Ashley Rice stated, "You don't have to be composed at all hours to be strong. You don't have to be bold [at all times] to be brave."[16] It will, however, demand that you become more creative, skillful, and crafty to be able to accomplish the things you once took for granted. You can still sparkle and shine your light bright for others to see without giving up on life and the little things you and I once enjoyed—dancing, singing, hobbies, or sports. It simply means that from now on, thanks to PD, we have to work at doing things differently to get the same results! This takes a little bit more concentration and stepping outside of our comfort zones . . . but we can still have every bit of fun as before and perhaps even a little bit more.

There is a certain freedom that comes from having a chronic illness where you have to reinvent yourself to make things work to your satisfaction. This is where your unique brand of personality, pizzazz, and artistic flair comes into play. I like to think of ourselves as being the salt that makes everything taste better and last longer.

Before you know it, you will be discovering new things and enjoying life to the fullest again! Trust me when I say that your children will love having a carefree, fun mom that knows how to roll with the punches. This teaches them flexibility and creativity as well. Your spouse will also appreciate you trying to keep everything together and spread your wings in the midst of PD. He will be inspired to be a better husband, father, and caregiver as the disease advances. When you experience days that are not so good, he and your family will know that being a little off kilter makes you no less beautiful, smart, or competent. It does not diminish your inner sparkle.

I began writing this book as a way of coping with this illness and also as a way to show women everywhere who struggle with this illness in their daily lives as patients, wives, mothers, daughters, caregivers that they, too, have the power within themselves to beat anything that is thrust their way—to show that Parkinson's in women is not our grandmother's disease and, thus, should not be treated as such. We are unique with individualized needs, expectations, desires, dreams, talents, and gifts. We as women are capable of so much more in this journey against PD than what we have allowed ourselves to believe.

But best of all, I want to stress the positive energy that empowers you and me to be able to crush Parkinson's comes from within, and the driving force comes from the fact that we are women. We are always ready for a challenge! To quote Audrey Hepburn, "Remember, if you ever need a helping hand, it's at the end of your arm, as you get older, remember you have another hand: The first to help yourself, the second is to help others."[12] By helping others, we, in turn, help ourselves to feel better and conquer our own fears and illness. But remember that in order to be an effective woman who cares for others, you must start by loving and caring for yourself FIRST! As a Nu Shu proverb goes, "The wise woman waters her own garden first."[13]

The first thing you must learn to do is love yourself, after God, in order to conquer the world and your illness. As fierce, strong PD women, we need to learn that there is nothing more powerful than standing in our own truth. This kind of confidence comes only after much introspection. Every morning before you do your facial exercises, take a good look at yourself in the mirror, and really look at the person staring back at you. I want you to notice your beauty, wrinkles and all, and search for the beauty that lies within, whether it is in your eyes or in your smile, and focus on your own gifts, talents, and qualities that are uniquely yours—then begin reciting your name out loud. Summon the diva within. As I have discovered, our name holds the key to our own personal destiny and inner fortitude. I personally don't like the shortened version of my full given name, which was given to me by my grandfather; thus, extremely special to me. All my important documents like my medical school diploma bear proudly my full given name. It matters what you call yourself. How you perceive yourself will influence how others perceive you. Remember, PD women may have more pronounced facies, which may bias even professionals into thinking that women with PD are depressed, and thus bias them against recommending certain treatment modalities like DBS, especially earlier in the disease. Thus, if you follow my tips of exercising your facial muscles daily with some added speech therapy to increase facial expression, along with reciting your name out loud in front of the mirror to help increase voice modulation, not only will it empower you as a woman to take charge over your life and PD, but this can potentially affect your mood and cognition in a positive manner.[14]

The shortened version of my name at times seems so commonplace to me, that when I engage in any activity I usually think of my nickname, which goes so much better with my DIVA persona. This much is true—within my family, my name or rather my nickname has become a verb, adjective, and a noun! It is absolutely true that "when you can say your name with pride for which you are, you will be the (most) powerful [PD] woman,"[15] capable of weathering any storm and conquering PD on your own terms. This means that you have unique skills and talents that can be refined, molded, reshaped, and even capable of acquiring new skills to fit the new life with Parkinson's we have been given. Unlike our grandmothers who had PD, we now have more resources and access to education and possibilities for vocational rehabilitation, which can allow us to continue to be independent in the face of a chronic illness, helping to relieve some of the mental anguish that comes along with having an uncertain financial future. Take care of your finances and your spiritual wellbeing; only then will you be able to blossom and emerge victorious and remain at peace while in the eye of the storm, even though all around you may seem like chaos.

So, next time before you get ready to go out, before you put on your favorite red lipstick, blue hat, purple running shoes or green scarf, look at yourself in the mirror and state your name out loud, boasting with confidence knowing that all the Parkinson's women around the world are standing right beside you. I look forward to the day we can all walk arm in arm at the Parkinson's Unity Walk, which is held in New York City in Central Park each spring, alongside other courageous women with PD—like my friends Peggy and Rhonda, who have pioneered changes in the way PD patients are perceived and treated; and Ruth Lotzer, the winner of the 2014 PDF T-shirt design and the "hope" pin.

Her beautifully crafted pin, which she graciously gifted me, serves as a daily reminder of the endless possibilities available to us women with PD if we just believe in ourselves. Individually and as a team, **we can make a difference in the fight against Parkinson's.**

Glossary

Frequently used Parkinson's terms

Bradykinesia: Greek term that means "slow movement" – it is one of the cardinal features of PD.

Basal ganglia: a series of interconnected regions of the brain including the striatum, globus pallidus, and thalamus.

Cogwheel rigidity: tension in a muscle that gives way in little jerks when it is passively stretched, one of the cardinal features of PD.

Dyskinesia: Greek for difficulty in movement, impairment in the ability to control movements resulting in fragmented or jerky movements.

Dose-related side effects (3 types):

1. Peak-dose dyskinesia: Occurs twenty to ninety minutes after taking medications (almost 75% of patients have them after six years of treatment; but in young patients, symptoms may occur before the end of the first year).

2. End-of-dose wearing-off phenomena: Effect of medication does not last from dose to dose. This is more common in patients with long-term therapy, correlated to low plasma concentrations of L-dopa and some may be due to interference of protein diet in absorption of medication.

3. Biphasic dose response: This is a phenomena where some patients experience dyskinesias of brief duration shortly after taking medication (especially first a.m. dose) which resolves only to be followed by onset of spasms and severe dystonia especially in lower extremities one to two hours later.

Dose-unrelated side effects: *On-off phenomena:* Occurs in 50% of patients that have been treated for five years or longer. These episodes consists of periods of unpredictable severe akinesia, hypotonia, and apprehension (anxiety) of very rapid onset and termination, which last from thirty minutes to a few hours and is unrelieved by further L-dopa dosing.

Dystonia: involuntary sustained contraction of muscles with increased muscle tone and resulting in abnormal posturing of muscles affected.

Globus pallidus: a portion of the basal ganglia affected in PD.

Hypophonia: soft voice/speech resulting from lack of coordination of vocal coordination.

Hypomimia: loss or impairment of facial expression.

Lee Silverman voice therapy: a method of training a person to strengthen his or her voice by singing loudly or shouting.

Micrographia: abnormally small, cramped handwriting and/or the progression to continually small handwriting.

Motor symptoms: the four main cardinal symptoms (slow movements, stiffness, loss of balance, and rest tremors) are collectively referred to as motor symptoms which make up Parkinsonism or the Parkinsonian syndrome, which are caused by loss of dopamine in the basal ganglia.

Non-motor symptoms: non-dopamine symptoms, i.e., RLS, constipation, loss of smell, hypotension, depression, anxiety, sexual dysfunction, hallucinations, bladder disorders, and psychosis.

Pallidotomy: a surgical procedure that can decrease dyskinesia, reduce tremor and improve bradykinesia.

Postural instability: loss of balance that causes someone to feel unsteady due to loss of postural reflexes, also a cardinal feature of PD.

Rest tremors: an involuntary coarse rhythmic tremor or quivering that consists of 3-5 hertz usually confined to the upper limbs of hands and forearms, present when arms are (relaxed) stretched at rest and disappear with activity or limbs become active. This is one of the four main cardinal features of PD-also described as "pill rolling."

Rigidity: inflexibility or stiffness due to increased muscle tone.

Thalamotomy: a surgical procedure targeting the thalamus designed to stop tremors.

Thalamus: portion of brain that receives sensory information.

Manual of neurologic Therapeutics 6th ed. Edited Samuels MA "Movement disorders." Lippincott Williams & Wilkins A Wolters Kluwer Company Philadelphia 1999. 15:375-383.

Lieberman A "100 Questions & Answers about Parkinson's Disease." (w. McCall M), Jones and Bartlett publishers, Sudbury, Mass. 2003. 225-230.

Organizations and Other Resources

Parkinson's Disease Foundation (PDF)
New York, NY
Info@pdf.org
18004576676
(212)923-4700
www.pdf.org

National Parkinson's Foundation (NPF)
Miami, FL
(800)327-4545
(800)473-4636
Contact@parkinson.org
www.parkinson.org

American Parkinson's Disease Association (APDA)
Staten Island, NY
(800)223-2732
Apda@apdaparkinson.org
www.apdaparkinson.org

Parkinson's Action Network (PAN)
Washington, DC
(800)850-4726
Info@parkinsonsaction.org
www.parkinsonsaction.org

Michael J. Fox Foundation for Parkinson's Research (MJFOX)
New York, NY
(800) 708-7644
info@michaeljfox.org
www.michaeljfox.org

Davis Phinney Parkinson's Foundation (DPF)
Boulder,CO
(866)358-0285
info@davisphinneyfoundation.org
www.davisphinneyfoundation.org

Muhammad Ali Parkinson's Center (MAPC)
The Barrow Neurological Institute of St. Joseph's Hospital and
Medical Center
Phoenix, Arizona
(602)406-6262

Movement Disorder Society
555 East Wells Street, Suite 1100
Milwaukee, WI 53202-3823
414-276-2145
info@movementdisorders.org

Houston Area Parkinson's Society
http://www.hapsonline.org/

Dallas Area Parkinson's Society
https://www.daps.us/

Depression
If you struggle with depression or suicide contact the National
Helpline of the Parkinson's Disease Foundation at (800) 457-6676

or via email at info@pdf.org. Or visit
http://www.suicidepreventionlifeline.org/www.Samaritans.org

Other Useful Websites for Caregivers
www.caregiving.org
www.caregiver.va.gov
www.caregiverstress.com
www.aarp.org/home-family/caregiving/
www.ecarediary.com
www.eldercare.gov
www.eldercarelink.com

Benefits of Massage Therapy
You can find out more information regarding this subject in a manual
called "Massage therapy: is it for you? Or by visiting www.parkinson.
org/Parkinson-s-Disease/PD-Library/NPF-publications which
provides a checklist on benefits of massage, etc.

Other Helpful Resources
Lieberman A, 100 Questions & Answers about Parkinson's Disease.
(w. McCall M), Jones and Bartlett Publishers, Sudbury, Mass. 2003.
225-230.

Parkinson's Disease Resource List, second edition PDF; 2011 Parkinson's Disease Foundation, Inc.
http://www.pdf.org/es/resourcelink/category/Driving
http://www.pdf.org/en/financial_planning financial assistance
http://www.pdf.org/en/legal_assistance_pdf
http://www.pdf.org/en/employ_concerns

About the Author

Maria De León is movement disorder neurologist, who completed her postgraduate fellowship training at Baylor College of Medicine in 1999. She was diagnosed with Parkinson's disease in 2008. Although she is currently on sabbatical, she spends her time involved in related activities as a well-respected and well-versed resource on PD. She is a consultant and frequent guest lecturer for the School of Social Work at Stephen F. Austin University; a member and research advocate for the People with

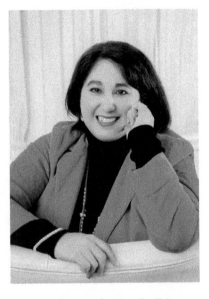

Parkinson's Advisory Committee (PPAC) for the Parkinson's Disease Foundation (PDF); and is the Texas assistant director for the Parkinson's Action Network (PAN).

Maria established www.defeatparkinsons.com along with one of her former Parkinson's patients, Howard A. "Woody" Wolfson. Since his passing, she now carries the full responsibility of running this organization, whose sole purpose is to provide free counseling to Parkinson's patients and their families in the East Texas region. She is also an active member of the Parkinson's Inside Out think tank, inaugurated in 2014. Concomitantly, she works vigorously to improve the lives of those with neurological disease at all levels by instructing pre-med students and health professionals alike. In 2013, she was the recipient of the Association of American University Women (AAUW) Award for her work in the field of medicine.

Parkinson's Diva: A Woman's Guide to Parkinson's Disease is a culmination of Maria's many experiences and insights. She resides with her husband and daughter in Nacogdoches, Texas. You can contact her through www.parkinsonsdiva.org, www.defeatparkinsons.com, and www.facebook.com/defeatparkinsons101.

References

Preface

1. Moyer, Melinda Wenner. "Drug Problem: Women aren't properly represented in scientific studies." http://www.slate.com/articles/health_and_science/medical_examiner/2010/07/drug_problem.html
2. Ibid.
3. Ibid.
4. Abott, Julie A., Women's Healthsource, Mayo Clinic.

Introduction: Facts & Demographics about Women

1. "Aging Trends Point to Business Opportunities" by Anthony Cirillo, About.com Guide
2. Ibid.
3. Canada has higher proportion of seniors than ever before. http://www.cbc.ca/news/canada/canada-has-higher-proportion-of-seniors-than-ever-before-1.1151526
4. Australian Demographic Statistics, Jun 2012 http://www.abs.gov.au/AUSSTATS/abs@.nsf/
1. "Aging Trends Point to Business Opportunities" by Anthony Cirillo, About.com Guide
2. Ibid.
3. Canada has higher proportion of seniors than ever before. http://www.cbc.ca/news/canada/canada-has-higher-proportion-of-seniors-than-ever-before-1.1151526
4. Australian Demographic Statistics, Jun 2012 http://www.abs.gov.au/AUSSTATS/abs@.nsf/featurearticlesbyCatalogue/541941F68CFBBB-30CA257B3B00117A34?OpenDocument
5. http://www.agediscrimination.info/statistics/Pages/CurrentUKpopulation.aspx
6. https://caregiver.org/women-and-caregiving-facts-and-figures

7. Ibid.

8. http://www.PDF.org/en/science_news/release/pr_1415296989)

9. Ibid.

Chapter 1: Parkinson's Women Improperly Represented in Clinical Studies

1. Moyer, Melinda Wenner. "Drug Problem: Women aren't properly represented in scientific studies." http://www.slate.com/articles/health_and_sci. ence/medical_examiner/2010/07/drug_problem.html

2. Migraine- more than a Headache. http://www.entad.org/docs/Migrainehandout.pdf

3. Moyer, Melinda Wenner. "Drug Problem: Women aren't properly represented in scientific studies." http://www.slate.com/articles/health_and_science/medical_examiner/2010/07/drug_problem.html

4. Diethylstilbestrol (DES) http://en.m.wikipedia.org/wiki/Diethylstilbestrol

5. Moyer, Melinda Wenner. "Drug Problem: Women aren't properly represented in scientific studies." http://www.slate.com/articles/health_and_science/medical_examiner/2010/07/drug_problem.html

6. Ibid.

7. Anxiety and Depression Association of America. "Pregnancy and medication." http://www.adaa.org/living-with-anxiety/women/pregnancy-and-medication

8. Moyer, Melinda Wenner. "Drug Problem: Women aren't properly represented in scientific studies." http://www.slate.com/articles/health_and_science/medical_examiner/2010/07/drug_problem.html

9. Ibid.

10. Ibid.

11. Martilla, R.J., Kaprio J., Konskenvuo M., and Rinne U.K. (Aug. 1988): Parkinson's disease in a nationwide twin cohort. Neurology 38(8):1217. Doi:10.1212/WNL.38.8.1217

12. Women in Academic Medicine Statistics and Medical school Benchmarking, 2011-2012. Figure 1: women as percentage of applicants to US Medical schools. https://www.aamc.org/members/gwims/statistics/stats12/

Chapter 2: History and Symptoms of Parkinson's Disease

1. Parkinson, J (2002). "An Essay on the Shaking Palsy. 1817." J. Neuropsychiatry Clin. Neurosci.14 (2):223—36; discussion 222. doi:10.1176/appi.neuropsych.14.2.223

2. http://en.m.wikipedia.org/wiki/History_of_Parkinson's_disease

3. Ibid.

4. Ibid.

5. Currier RD (April 1996). "Did John Hunter Give James Parkinson an Idea?' Arch. Neurol. 53(4): 377-8.

6. Garcia Ruiz PJ (December 2004). "Prehistoria de la enfermedad de Parkinson." [Prehistory of Parkinson's disease]. Neurologia (in Spanish Castillian) 19(10): 735-7.

7. http://en.m.wikipedia.org/wiki/History_of_Parkinson's_disease

8. Ibid.

9. "A History of Parkinson's Disease". https://www.atrainceu.com/course-module/1874198-080_antiparkinson-strategies-module-01

10. Goetz, CG. (September 2011): "The History of Parkinson's Disease: Early Clinical Descriptions and Neurological Therapies." Cold Spring Harb Perspect Med 1(1):1-27)

11. Katzenschlger R, Evans A, et al. (2004). "Mucuna pruriens in Parkinson's disease: a double blind clinical and pharmacological study." J. Neurol Neurosurg Psychiatry 75 (12):1672-1677. doi:10.1136/jnnp.2003.028761

12. Ibid.

13. https://nwpf.org/stay-informed/blog/2013/07/is-natural-dopamine-better-than-sinemet/

14. Ibid.

15. Chaudhuri, RK.(March 2014): "Under-recognized non-motor symptoms of Parkinson's Disease." PDF Expert Briefings.

16. http://en.m.wikipedia.org/wiki/History_of_Parkinson's_disease

17. Focus on Parkinson's Disease. "Levodopa: Is Toxicity a Myth?" http://www.epda.eu.com/EasysiteWeb/getresource. axd?AssetID=16292&type=full&servicetype=Attachment

18. / http://www.pdf.org/en/science_news/release/pr_1365719110

19. Focus on Parkinson's Disease. "Levodopa: Is Toxicity a Myth?" http://www.epda.eu.com/EasysiteWeb/getresource. axd?AssetID=16292&type=full&servicetype=Attachment

20. Dorsey ER, Constantinescu R., Thompson JP et al. (2007) Projected

number of people with Parkinson's disease in the most populous nations, 2005 through 2030. Neurology 68(5):384-386.

21. Pavon, JM, Whitson, HE, Okun, MS., (April 2010) "Parkinson's disease in women: A call for improved clinical studies and for comparative effectiveness research." Maturitas 65(4):352-358.

Chapter 3: Parkinson's Disease Presentation Varies Depending on Age of Onset and Gender

1. Moyer, Melinda Wenner. "Drug Problem: Women aren't properly represented in scientific studies." http://www.slate.com/articles/health_and_science/medical_examiner/2010/07/drug_problem.html

2. "Migraine: More than a Headache." http://www.entad.org/docs/Migrainehandout.pdf

3. http://www.everydayhealth.com/health-report/major-depression/depression-statistics.aspx

4. Bonnet AM, Jutras MF, Czernecki V, et. Al. (2012) Review article: Nonmotor Symptoms in Parkinson's Disease in 2012: Relevant Clinical Aspects http://dx.doiorg/10.1155/2012/198316

5. http://www.pdf.org/pdf/parkinson_briefing_nontmotor_slides_031113.pdf

6. "Fatigue in early Parkinson's Disease." (March 2012) Science News. http://www.pdf.org/en/science_news/release/pr_1331222820

7. http://www.youngparkinsons.org/.../articles/is-pain-a-symptom-of-parkinsons-disease

8. Bonnet AM, Jutras MF, Czernecki V, et. Al. (2012) Review article: Nonmotor Symptoms in Parkinson's Disease in 2012: Relevant Clinical Aspects http://dx.doiorg/10.1155/2012/198316

9. "Fatigue in Early Parkinson's Disease." (March 2012): Science News. http://www.pdf.org/en/science_news/release/pr_1331222820

10. Noonan D. (May 2014): "Inside the science of an amazing new surgery called Deep Brain Stimulation: the most futuristic medical treatment ever imagined is now a reality." Smithsonian Magazine 1-2. http://www.smithsonianmag.com/innovation/inside-science-amazing-new-surgery-called-deep-brain-stimulation-180951170/?no-ist=&fb_locale=ar_AR&page=2

11. GOETZ CG. (AUG. 2009): "JEAN MARTIN CHARCOT AND HIS VIBRATORY CHAIR FOR PARKINSON'S DISEASE. NEUROLOGY 73(6):475-478.

12. http://www.etymonline.com/index.php?term=thalamus

13. Noonan D. (May 2014): "Inside the science of an amazing new surgery called Deep Brain Stimulation: the most futuristic medical treatment ever imagined is now a reality." Smithsonian Magazine 1-2. http://www.smithsonianmag.com/innovation/inside-science-amazing-new-surgery-called-deep-brain-stimulation-180951170/?no-ist=&fb_locale=ar_AR&page=2

14. Science News (Jan 2014) "Studies Find Disparities in Use of Deep Brain Stimulation." http://www.pdf.org/en/science_news/release/pr_1391019029

15. Focus on Parkinson's disease. "Levodopa: Is Toxicity a Myth?" http://www.epda.eu.com/EasysiteWeb/getresource.axd?AssetID=16292&type=full&servicetype=Attachment

16. Marras Connie MD, PhD, and Saunders-Pullman Rachel M, MPH (June 2014) "Complexities of hormonal influences and risk of PD" Mov Disord 29 (7):845-848

17. Pavon, JM, Whitson, HE, Okun, MS., (April 2010) "Parkinson's disease in women: A call for improved clinical studies and for comparative effectiveness research." Maturitas 65(4):352-358.

18. http://www.healthline.com/health-slideshow/parkinsons-symtoms-men-women

19. Ibid.

20. Science News (May 2014) : "Parkinson's Disease Symptoms Vary with Age of Disease Onset." http://www.pdf.org/en/science_news/release/pr_1399644766

21. Liu R., Baird Donna, Park Yikyung et al. (June 2014) "Female reproductive factors, menopausal hormone use, and Parkinson's disease." Mov disord 29 (7):889-896

22. Marras C. and Saunders-Pullman R. (June 2014) "Complexities of hormonal influences and risk of PD" Mov Disord 29 (7):845-848

23. Marras C. and Saunders-Pullman R. (June 2014) "Complexities of hormonal influences and risk of PD" Mov Disord 29 (7):845-848

24. Rossouw J, Prentice R. Manson J, et al. (2007): "Postmenopausal hormone therapy and risk of cardiovascular disease by age and years since menopause." J Am Med Assoc 297:1465-1477.

25. Maki P. (2013): 'Critical Window Hypothesis of Hormone Therapy and Cognition: a scientific Update on Clinical Studies.' Menopause 20:695-709.

26. Sherwin B. (2009): 'Estrogen Therapy is Time of Initiation Critical for Neuroprotection?' Nat Rev Endocrinol 5:620:-627.

27. Suzuki S, Brown C, Dela Cruz C, et al. (2007): "Timing of estrogen therapy after ovariectomy dictates the efficacy of its neuroprotective and antiinflamatory actions. *Pro Natl Acad Sci USA* 104:6013-6018.

28. Demirkian M, Aslan K, Bicakci S, et al. (2004): 'Transient parkinsonism: Induced by progesterone or pregnancy?' *Mov Disord* 19(11):1382-1384.

29. Scott M, Chowdhury M. (2005): 'Pregnancy in Parkinson's disease; unique case report and review of the literature.' *Mov Disord* 20(8):1078-1079.

30. Pavon, JM, Whitson, HE, Okun, MS., (April 2010) "Parkinson's disease in women: A call for improved clinical studies and for comparative effectiveness research." *Maturitas* 65(4):352-358.

31. Symptoms of Parkinson's of men vs. women –Healthline http://www.healthline.com/health-slideshow/parkinsons-symptoms-men-women

32. Nazario B. (June 2005): "Why Men & Women Handle Stress Differently." http://www.webmd.com/women/features/stress-women-men-cope

33. Nazario B. (June 2005): "Why Men & Women Handle Stress Differently." http://www.webmd.com/women/features/stress-women-men-cope

34. Science News (May 2014) : "Parkinson's disease Symptoms Vary with age of Disease Onset" http://www.pdf.org/en/science_news/release/pr_1399644766

35. Depression in women understanding the gender gap –Mayo Clinic http://www.mayoclinic.org/diseases-conditions/depression/in-depth/depression/art-20047725

36. http://www.empr.com/depression-in-neurological-disease/article/283884

37. *Goleman Daniel(Dec 1990): Women's depression rate is higher:* http://www.nytimes.com/1990/12/06/health/women-s-depression-rate-is-higher.html

38. Women in parkinson's disease understanding the specific journey: http://www.pdf.org/fall14_women_parkinson

39. Liu R., Baird Donna, Park Yikyung et al. (June 2014) "Female reproductive factors, menopausal hormone use, and Parkinson's disease." *Mov disord* 29 (7):889-896

40. Okun MS. (Feb 2012): 'Post of the week: High Hip Fracture rate in Parkinson's disease.' http://forum.parkinson.org/index.php?/topic/12297-post-of-the-week-high-hip-fracture-rate-in-parkinsons-disease/

41. Parkinson's Disease Foundation (2009): 'Low Vitamin D levels Associated with Parkinson's Disease.' *News & Review*

42. Walker RW, Chaplain A, Hancock RL, et.al. (March 2013): 'Hip Fractures in people with idiopathic Parkinson's disease: incidence and outcomes.' Mov Disord 28(3):334-40. doi.1002/mds.25297. Epub2013 Feb 6.

43. Parkinson's Disease Foundation (2009): 'Low Vitamin D levels Associated with Parkinson's Disease.' *News & Review*

44. Okun MS. (Feb 2012): 'Post of the week: High Hip Fracture rate in Parkinson's disease.' http://forum.parkinson.org/index.php?/topic/12297-post-of-the-week-high-hip-fracture-rate-in-parkinsons-disease/

45. Women's healthsource Mayo Clinic desk of Julie A. Abott medical director page 1

Chapter 4: Misdiagnosing PD in Young Women

1. Garcia de Andrade LC (Dec 1996): "A comprehensive critical review on early onset Parkinson's disease." Arquivos de Neuro-Psiqiatria (Spanish Archives of Neuro-Psychiatry) 54(4):691-704. Doi:10.1590/S0004-282X19960000400024

2. Kittle G. "Parkinson Disease: what you and your family should know." 3rd ed. National Parkinson Foundation

3. "Environmental factors and Parkinson's: what have we learned?" PDF http://www.pdf.org/environment_parkinsons_tanner

4. Adamson J, Ben-Shlomo Y, Chaturvedi N, et al. (2003): "Ethnicity, socio-economic position and gender—do they affect reported healthcare-seeking behavior?" Soc Sci Med 57:895-904.

5. Saunders-Pullman R, Wang C, Bressman SB. (June 2011): "Diagnosis and referral delay in women with Parkinson's Disease." Gend Med 8(3):209-217.

6. Chaudhuri RK, Prieto-Jurcynska C, Naidu Y, et al (2010): "the non-declaration of non-motor symptoms of Parkinson's disease to healthcare professionals. An international study using non-motor questionnaire." Mov Disord 25(6):704-709.

7. Female hysteria. en.wikipedia.org/wiki/Female_hysteria

8. Hysteria. en.wikipedia.org/wiki/Hysteria

9. "Epilepsy: from the early civilizations to modern days." http://www.hektoeninternational.org/index.php?option=com_content&view=article&id=1175

10. Owens C and Dein S. "Conversion disorder: the modern hysteria." Advances in psychiatric treatment. http://apt.rcpsych.org/content/12/2/152.full

11. Ibid.

12. Ibid.

13. "Primary torsion dystonia." http://emedicine.medscape.com/article/1150643-overview

14. Swain JE, Leckman JF. (July 2005): "Tourette syndrome and tic disorders." Psychiatry (Edgmont) 2(7):26-36.

15. Lakhan S and Viera KF "Schizophrenia pathophysiology: are we any closer to a complete model? " http://www.annals-general-psychiatery.com/content/8/1/12

16. "Parkinson's disease among Hispanics and whites." http://anthropology.msu.edu/anp204-us12/2012/07/13/parkinsons-disease-among-hispanics-and-whites/

17. " Americans in 2020: less whites, more southern." (April 1994): http://www.nytimes.com/1994/04/22/us/americans-in-2020-less-white-more-southern.html

18. Szasz T. (May 2011): "The Second Sin." http://www.quotegarden.com/medical.html

19. Chaudhuri RK.(March 2014):"Under Recognized non-motor symptoms of Parkinson's Disease." PDF Expert Briefings.

20. Haughn Z. (March 2014): Movement disorder Focus with the Michael J Fox Foundation. "Thinking outside the Brain-Alpha synuclein pathology linked to Parkinson's is being detected outside the brain, in places like the salivary glands, retina and colon." Practical Neurology 26-28.

21. Ibid.

Chapter 5: Coping with Parkinson's: Spirituality, Religion & Health

1. Axelrod J. (Dec 2014) :"5 stages of loss and grief." http://psychcentral.com/lib/the-5-stages-of-loss-and-grief/000617

2. Faith. King James Bible " authorized version," Cambridge edition Hebrews 11:1

3. Brenner CB, and Zacks JM. (Dec 2011): why walking through a doorway makes you forget." Scientific American

4. Guibert S. (Nov 2011): "Walking through doorways causes forgetting, new research shows" Notre Dame News

5. Parkinson-Northcote C. "Delay is deadliest is the deadliest form of denial." Brainy Quote. http://www.brainyquote.com/quotes/quotes/c/cnorthcot159773.html

6. Plato.http://www.science20.com/scientist/blog/physician_quotes-64984

7. Plato quote. "You ought not attempt to cure the body without the soul." Notable quotes. http://www.notable-quotes.com/p/plato_quotes_ii.html

8. Reber, W. (1900) JAMA. Cited by Cohen, "JJ in the healing as art: Integrating humanism in the medical school curriculum." AAMC Reporter 9(12):1. September, 2000.

9. Chez RA and Jonas Wayne B. "Proceedings: Spiritual transformation and health through the lifecycle: Meditation and spirituality for healthcare providers."

10. Copp Jay. (March 2000): "Faith and Medicine: A growing Practice" Issue of St. Anthony Messenger. http://www.americancatholic.org/Messenger?Mar2000/feature2.asp

11. Ibid.

12. Ibid.

13. Ibid.

14. Ibid

15. Baime M. (July 2011): "This is your brain on mindfulness." Shambhala Sun 45-84. http://www.3D4Medical.com/science photo library

16. Ibid.

17. Ibid.

18. Brain benefits of practicing mindfulness meditation http://askdrdani.com/brain-benefits-of-practicing-mindfulness-meditation/

19. Copp Jay. (March 2000): "Faith and Medicine: A growing Practice" Issue of St. Anthony Messenger. http://www.americancatholic.org/Messenger?Mar2000/feature2.asp

20. Kosmin B and Keysar A (2009): "Data from ARIS-American Religious Identification Survey- 2008." Hartford CT: Trinity College http://www.americanreligionsurvey-aris.org/

21. Glaquinto S, Bruti L, Dall'Armi V et al. (2011): Religious and spiritual beliefs in outpatients suffering from Parkinson Disease. International Journal of Geriatric Psychiatry 26(9): 916-922.

22. Balanger K. (March 2012): 'Religion, spirituality and health." Parkinson's symposium SFA University.

23. Koening HG (2007): "Religion and depression in older medical inpatients." American Journal of Geriatric Psychiatry 15(4):282-291.

24. Koening HG (2007): "Religion and remission of depression in medical patients with heart failure/pulmonary disease." Journal of Nervous and Mental Disease 195:000-000.

25. Gass B. (2009): "The Best of the word for you today: 365 days of strength and guidance: above and beyond." 5: (April5).

26. Hummer R, Rogers R, Nam C, and Ellison C. (1999): "Religious involvement and US adult mortality." Demography 36: 273-285.

27. Hermann M, Curio N, Petz T. et al (2000): Coping with illness after brain diseases: a comparison between patients with malignant tumors, stroke, Parkinson's disease and traumatic brain injury. Disability & Rehabilitation 22(12):539-546.

28. Spirituality and spiritual wellbeing. EPDA. http://www.epda.eu.com/en/parkinsons/in-depth/managing-your-parkinsons/daily-living/spirituality-and-spiritual-wellbeing/

29. OLIPHANT E. AND CORDOVA W. (JANUARY 2015): "HIV AND WOMEN OF COLOR IN EAST TEXAS: TECHNIQUES TO ADDRESS CULTURAL BARRIERS."

30. Balanger K. (March 2012): 'Religion, spirituality and health." Parkinson's symposium SFA University.

Chapter: 6: Raising Children When Mom Has Parkinson's

1. PDF News & Review (Spring 2012): Seeking out a Parkinson's Specialist.

2. Muhammad Ali quotes. https://www.goodreads.com/quotes/90324-champions-aren-t-made-in-gyms-champions-are-made-from-something

Here are some books which may help you as parents or grandparents broach the topic with your children. Read them together and talk about them. These are some of mine and daughter's favorite books on PD (ages: toddlers to young teens)

Who is Pee Dee? – Explaining Parkinson's Disease to a Child by Kay Mixon Jenkins (www.whoispeedee.com)

Monica, Mama, and the Ocotillo's Leaves, by Adele P. Hensley (www.thewordverve.com/ocotillo)

I'll Hold Your Hand So You Won't Fall: A Child's Guide to Parkinson's Disease, by Rasheda Ali (www.meritpublishing.com)
How Marty's Mom Became a Cyborg, by Adele P. Hensley (www.thewordverve.com/cyborg)

My Grandpa's Shaky Hands by Soania Mathur

Chapter 7: Pregnancy and PD: What to Expect When You Are Expecting?

1. Rubin SM. "Parkinson's Disease in women: What you should know about early onset Parkinson's disease." http://www.youngparkinsons.org/what-you-should-know-about-early-onset-parkinsons-disease/articles/parkinsons-disease-in-women

2. California PD Registry http://www.capdregistry.org/

3. Nebraska PD Registry http://dhhs.ne.gov/publichealth/Pages/ced_parkinsons_index.aspx

4. Rubin SM. "Parkinson's Disease in women: What you should know about early onset Parkinson's disease." http://www.youngparkinsons.org/what-you-should-know-about-early-onset-parkinsons-disease/articles/parkinsons-disease-in-women

5. Ibid.

6. Menstruation and menopause. EPDA. http://www.epda.eu.com/en/parkinsons/in-depth/managing-your-parkinsons/daily-living/women-parkinsons/menstruation-menopause/

7. Yadav R., Shukla G., Goyal V., Singh S., and Behari M. (Aug 2012): "A case control of women with Parkinson's disease and their fertility characteristics." J Neurol Sci 319(1-2):135-138. Doi:10.1016/j.jns.2012.05.026. Epub2012 May 28

8. Scott M, Chowdhury M. (2005): 'Pregnancy in Parkinson's disease; unique case report and review of the literature.' Mov Disord 20(8):1078-1079.

9. Demirkian M, Aslan K, Bicakci S, et al. (2004): "Transient parkinsonism: Induced by progesterone or pregnancy?" Mov Disord 19(11):1382-1384.

10. Rubin SM. "Parkinson's Disease in women: What you should know about early onset Parkinson's disease." http://www.youngparkinsons.org/what-you-should-know-about-early-onset-parkinsons-disease/articles/parkinsons-disease-in-women

11. Ibid.

12. Miyasaki, JM, AlDakheel A. (Feb 2014): "Movement disorder of Pregnancy: RLS." Continuum 20 (1): 148-149.

13. Earley CJ. (2003): 'Clinical practice. Restless legs syndrome.' N Engl J Med 348(21):2103-2109.

14. Chesson AL Jr. et al. (1999): "Practice parameters for the treatment of restless leg syndrome and periodic limb movement disorder." Sleep 22(7):961-968.

15. Miyasaki, JM, AlDakheel A. (Feb 2014): "Movement disorder of pregnancy: RLS." Continuum 20(1):149.

16. Chesson AL Jr. et al. (1999): "Practice parameters for the treatment of restless leg syndrome and periodic limb movement disorder." Sleep 22(7):961-968.

17. Miyasaki, JM, AlDakheel A. (Feb 2014): "Movement disorder of pregnancy: RLS." Continuum 20(1):149.

18. Schuepbach WMM, Rau J, Knudsen K, Volkmann J, et al. (Feb 2013): 'Neurostimulation for Parkinsons Disease with early motor complications." N Engl J Med 368:610-622. http://www.nejm.org/doi/full/10.1056/NEJMoa1205158

19. Paluzzi A : "Pregnancy in dystonic women with in situ deep brain stimulators." http://www.researchgate.net/publication/7487519_Pregnancy_in_dystonic_women_with_in_situ_deep_brain_stimulators

20. Paluzzi A et al. (2006): "DBS in movement disorders-pregnancy." http://www.medmerits.com/index.php/article/deep_brain_stimulation_in_movement_disorders/P11

21. Miyasaki JM, AlDakheel A. (February 2014): 'Movement disorders in Pregnancy: Parkinsonism.' Continuum 20 (1): 155-156.

Chapter 8: Love and Marriage in PD (Until Death Do Us Part)

1. Gass B. (2009): "The Best of the word for you today: 365 days of strength and guidance: above and beyond: Debunking marriage myths (4)." 5(May15).

2. http://www.ncbi.nlm.nih.gov/pmc/articles/PMC1779554/

3. Divorce rate among MS and spine-injury patients. https://books.google.com/books?id=D6lYO_28vBEC&pg=PA179&lpg=PA179&d-q=divorce+rates+among+ms+and+spine+injury&source=bl&ots=W-B57h9avp9&sig=yKY1sbXAleGDd0zXKeNp928DRSQ&hl=en&sa=X-&ei=EyCgVPqBLcmlNtu4g9AO&ved=0CC8Q6AEwBzgK#v=onep-age&q=divorce%20rates%20among%20ms%20and%20spine%20inju-ry&f=false

4. Kilborn. P T. (May 1999): "Disabled spouses are increasingly forced to go at it alone." New York Times health. http://www.nytimes.com/1999/05/31/us/disabled-spouses-are-increasingly-forced-to-go-it-alone.html

5. Ibid.

6. Two myths and three facts about the differences in men and women's brains. http://www.psychologytoday.com/blog/brain-myths/201207/two-myths-and-three-facts-about-the-differences-in-men-and-womens-brains

7. Parker-Pope T. "Divorce risk higher when wife gets sick." http://well.blogs.nytimes.com/2009/11/12/men-more-likely-to-leave-spouse-with-cancer/?_r=0

8. Ibid.

9. Ibid.

10. Divorce rates are high in patients with MS, PD, and brain cancer. http://neurotalk.psychcentral.com/showthread.php?t=45140

11. Land Before Time lyrics, "You Are One of Us Now." http://www.lyricsmania.com/you_are_one_of_us_now_lyrics_land_before_time_the.html

12. Nambi S. (Jan-Mar 2005): "Marriage, mental health, and the Indian legislation." Indian Journal of Psychiatry 47(1):3-14.

Chapter 9: Sex and Parkinson's: The Bedroom Goddess

1. Henry Louis Mencken quotes on sexuality. http://www.quotes.net/quote/15600

2. Bronner G. (Sep 2013): "PD Expert Briefing :Sexuality and intimacy in Parkinson's." http://www.pdf.org/pdf/parkinson_briefing_sex_slides_091013.pdf

3. Rettner R. (April 2012):"Parkinson's personality: disease more likely to strike cautious people." MyHealthNewsDaily. http://www.livescience.com/20008-parkinsons-disease-personality-risk-avoidance.html

4. Sex sensuality intimacy and PD. EPDA. http://www.epda.eu.com/en/parkinsons/in-depth/managing-your-parkinsons/daily-living/women-parkinsons/intimacy-sexuality/

5. Bronner G. (Sep 2013): "PD Expert Briefing: Sexuality and intimacy in Parkinson's." http://www.pdf.org/pdf/parkinson_briefing_sex_slides_091013.pdf

6. Ibid.

7. Sex sensuality intimacy and PD. EPDA. http://www.epda.eu.com/en/parkinsons/in-depth/managing-your-parkinsons/daily-living/women-parkinsons/intimacy-sexuality/

8. Brain sex in men and women, from arousal to orgasm. http://brainblogger.com/2014/05/20/brain-sex-in-men-and-women-from-arousal-to-orgasm/

9. Lindau ST, Schumm LP, Laumann EO et al. (Aug 2007): "A study of sexuality and health among older adults in the United States." N Eng J Med 357(8):762-774.

10. Helgason AR, Adolfsson J, Dickman P et al. (1996): "Sexual desire, erection, orgasm and ejaculatory functions and their importance to elderly Swedish men: A population-based study." Age Ageing 25:285-291.

11. Freeman, Shanna. "What happens in the brain during an orgasm?" http://health.howstuffworks.com/sexual-health/sexuality/brain-during-orgasm2.htm

12. Antonovsky H, sadowsky M, Maoz B. (1990): "Sexual activity of aging men and women: an Israeli study." Behav Health Aging 3:151-161.

13. Bronner G. (Sep 2013): "PD Expert Briefing :Sexuality and intimacy in Parkinson's." http://www.pdf.org/pdf/parkinson_briefing_sex_slides_091013.pdf

14. Ibid.

15. Intimacy and sexuality. http://www.epda.eu.com/en/parkinsons/in-depth/managing-your-parkinsons/daily-living/women-parkinsons/intimacy-sexuality/

16. Science News (May 2014) : "Parkinson's Disease Symptoms Vary with Age of Disease Onset" http://www.pdf.org/en/science_news/release/pr_1399644766

17. Intimacy and sexuality. http://www.epda.eu.com/en/parkinsons/in-depth/managing-your-parkinsons/daily-living/women-parkinsons/intimacy-sexuality/

18. Bronner G. (Sep 2013): "PD Expert Briefing: Sexuality and intimacy in Parkinson's." http://www.pdf.org/pdf/parkinson_briefing_sex_slides_091013.pdf

19. Science News (May 2014) : "Parkinson's Disease Symptoms Vary with Age of Disease Onset" http://www.pdf.org/en/science_news/release/pr_1399644766

20. Frohman EM. (2002): "Sexual dysfunction in neurological disease." Clin Neuropharmacol 25:126-132.

21. Rutlen Richardson, Carmen. (2004): "Dancing Naked. . . in fuzzy red slippers." Cypress House. 71.

22. Ibid.

23. Hackney ME, BFA, and Earhart GM. (May 2009): "Effects of dance on movement control in Parkinson's disease: a comparison of Argentine Tango and American ballroom." J Rehabil Med 41(6):475-481.

24. www.victoriassecret.com

Recommended media:

Awakenings by Oliver Sacks

Movie: *Love & Other Drugs*

Chapter 10: Parkinson Medication Effect on the Female Patient

1. Moyer, Melinda Wenner. "Drug Problem: Women aren't properly represented in scientific studies." http://www.slate.com/articles/health_and_science/medical_examiner/2010/07/drug_problem.html

2. "10 incredible facts about the criminal mind." http://www.criminaljusticedegreesguide.com/features/10-incredible-facts-about-the-criminal-brain.html

3. Baskerville T, Douglas AJ. (Jun 2010): "Dopamine and oxytocin interactions underlying behaviors: potential contributions to behavioral disorders." CNS Neurosci Ther 16(3): e92-123. Doi.10.1111/j.1755-5949.2010.00154.x.

4. Ibid.

5. Weintraub D. (Sep 2011): "Impulsive and compulsive Behaviors in Parkinson's PDF Expert Brief." http://www.pdf.org/en/parkinson_briefing_impulsive_behaviors

6. "Woman's spontaneous orgasm triggered by Parkinson's drug.".http://www.livescience.com/47208-spontaneous-orgasms-parkinsons-drug-rasagiline.html

7. Vohra A. (Oct 2012): "Treatment of multiple distressing spontaneous orgasms with citalopram and their re-emergence following discontinuation of prolonged use of citalopram in an adult female survivor of child sexual abuse." Indian J Psychiatry 54(4):378-380. http://www.ncbi.nlm.nih.gov/pmc/articles/PMC3554973/

8. Ibid.

9. Krans B. (Sep 2012): Reviewed Kruck G. :Orgasmic dysfunction causes, symptoms & diagnosis http://www.healthline.com/health/orgasmic-dysfunction#Treatment5

10. "Woman's spontaneous orgasm triggered by Parkinson's drug.".http://www.livescience.com/47208-spontaneous-orgasms-parkinsons-drug-rasagiline.html

11. Ibid.

12. Ibid.

13. Menstruation and menopause. EPDA. http://www.epda.eu.com/en/
    parkinsons/in-depth/managing-your-parkinsons/daily-living/women-
    parkinsons/menstruation-menopause/

14. Ibid.

15. "Migraine: More than a headache." ahttp://fox6now.com/2014/09/17/
    migraines-with-aura-in-middle-age-linked-to-parkinsons-disease/

16. "Link between migraine and Parkinson's." Medical News Today http://
    www.medicalnewstoday.com/articles/282678.php

17. Ibid.

18. Definition of penetrance. http://en.m.wikipedia.org/wiki/Penetrance

19. "Link found between migraine and Parkinson's." Medical News Today
    http://www.medicalnewstoday.com/articles/282678.php

20. http://doublecheckmd.com/EffectsDetail.
    do?dname=Azilect&sid=70623&eid=2435

21. www.womenshealthmag.com/. . . /bacterial-vaginosis-gardnerella-vaginitis

22. http://doublecheckmd.com/EffectsDetail.
    do?dname=Azilect&sid=70623&eid=2435

23. Kim, Ja-Hong. (September 2014): "Management of Overactive Bladder
    and Urge Incontinence." Practical Neurology. 13(7): 27-32.

24. UTI prevention. http://www.upmc.com/patients-visitors/education/
    womens-health/pages/urinary-tract-infection.aspx

25. "Higher rates of certain cancers among LRRK2 gene mutation carriers
    with PD." (Dec 2014): Science News. http://www.pdf.org/en/science_
    news/release/pr_1418740778

Chapter 11: Beauty Tips for the Parkinson's Diva

1. Suzy Toronto http://suzytoronto.com/words-to-live-by/category/listing

2. http://scienceblogs.com/neurophilosophy/2010/04/16/botox-may-
   diminish-the experience-of-emotions/

3. http://www.researchgate.net/publication/35919406_Diminished_
   affective_modulation_of_startle_to_threatening_stimuli_in_
   parkinson%27s_disease_electronic_resource_

4. Ibid.

5. Pluck, GC and Brown RG (July 2002):"Apathy in Parkinson's disease." J Neurol Neurosurg Psychiatry73:636-642 doi:10.1136/jnnp.73.6.636

6. Alves, G, Forsaa EB, Pedersen KF, Gjerstad MD, Larsen JP (2008): J Neurol "Epidemiology of Parkinson's disease." 255(Suppl 5: 18-32. Doi10.1007/s00415-008-5004-3

7. Audrey Hepburn quote. http://www.curatedquotes.com/audrey-hepburn-quotes/

8. Maria Shapova quote. http://www.brainyquote.com/quotes/quotes/m/mariashara433691.html

9. Rutlen CR. "Dancing Naked ...in fuzzy red slippers." Cypress House 2004 pg. 163

10. http://www.empower-yourself-with-color-psycology.com/color-white.html

11. http://www.empower-yourself-with-colorpsychology.com/color-black.html

12. Audrey Hepburn quote. http://www.curatedquotes.com/audrey-hepburn-quotes/

13. "The Japanese Art of Kintsugi." https://www.google.com/?gws_rd=ssl#q=japanese+art+using+gold+to+fill+broken+parts

Chapter 12: Tools & Gadgets Every Parkinson's Diva Should Own

1. National Parkinson's foundation for info on kitchen and bathroom and apps http://www.parkinson.org/Parkinson-s-Disease/Living-Well/Safety-at-Home/Kitchen-Safety-Tips

2. Meed C. "The meaning of color: choosing a color palette for your home." http://EzineArticles.com/?expert=Collin_Meed

3. http://www.empower-yourself-with-color-psychology.com-brown.html

4. http://www.npr.org/blogs/health/2014/05/13/310399325/a-spoon-that-shakes-to-counteract-hand-tremors

5. "The 5 healing effects of lavender." Health.com http://www.health.com/health/gallery/0,,20587573,00.html

6. "A cold splash: hydrotherapy for depression and anxiety." Psychology Today. http://www.psychologytoday.com/blog/inner-source/201407/cold-splash-hydrotherapy-depression-and-anxiety

7. Hippocrates and the Water Cure: http://www.watercure2.org/hippocrates. htm

8. van Tubergen A, van der Linden S. (2002): "A brief history of spa therapy." Ann Rheum Dis 61:273-275. Doi. 10.1136/ard.61.3.273.

9. "A cold splash: hydrotherapy for depression and anxiety." Psychology Today. http://www.psychologytoday.com/blog/inner-source/201407/cold-splash-hydrotherapy-depression-and-anxiety

10. http://allgaragefloors.com/best-garage-parking-aids/

11. http://seniordriving.aaa.com/

12. iPhone apps. http://www.apppicker.com/applists/10599/The-best-iPhone-apps-for-Parkinsons

13. Life vac: https://lifevac.net/

Chapter 13: Domestic Diva and PD

1. Why your brain craves music http://science.time.com/2013/04/15/music/

Chapter 14: What Every Woman with Parkinson's Should Have

1. Orman S. (2007): "Women & Money: owning the power to control your destiny." Spiegel & Grau New York. pg. 31

2. Ibid. pg32

3. Di Vincenzo M. (2012) "Buy Shoes on Wednesday and tweet at 4:00: Getting the Job Done." 8:113.

4. Di Vincenzo M. (2012) "Buy Shoes on Wednesday and tweet at 4:00: Getting Rich." 6:77.

5. Imke S, Hutton T, and Loftus S. Parkinson Disease: Caring and Coping. National Parkinson Foundation. 46-47.

6. Di Vincenzo M. (2012) "Buy Shoes on Wednesday and tweet at 4:00: Getting Rich." 6:77.

7. Imke S, Hutton T, and Loftus S. Parkinson Disease: Caring and Coping. National Parkinson Foundation. 46-47.

Chapter 15: Four keys to Unlocking Happiness in the Midst of PD

1. PD personality http://www.livescience.com/20008-parkinsons-disease-personality-risk-avoidance.html

2. "Prevalence of Parkinson's disease." http://viartis.net/parkinsons.disease/
    prevalence.htm
3. http://en.m.wikipedia.org/wiki/Neurobiological_effects_of_physical_
    exercise
4. Gass B. (2009): "The best of the word for you today-365 days of strength
    and guidance: happiness Key (2)." Vol 5. January 27.

Chapter 16: Exercise and PD

1. 1.Gass B. (1996): "Best of the Word for today: Paganini's violin" April 4
    pg.95
2. 2.Ibid.
3. 3.Ibid.
4. 4 Knekt P, Kikkinen A, Rissanen H et al. (July 2010): Serum vitamin D
    and the risk of Parkinson Disease." Arch Neurol 67(7):808-811. Doi:
    10.1001/archneurol.2010.120.
5. "The human brain –exercise." http://www.fi.edu/learn/brain/exercise.html
    1-16.
6. Ibid. pg12
7. Ibid. pg 16
8. Ibid. pg 14
9. Ibid.
10. Ibid.
11. Could brisk walking be therapeutic for people with Parkinson's? Medical
    News Today http://www.medicalnewstoday.com/articles/279085.php
12. Painting rainbow. http://www.everyday-taichi.com/taiji-qigong.html#sh3
13. "The human brain, an exercise." http://www.fi.edu/learn/brain/exercise.
    html 1-16.

Chapter 17: Emotional exhaustion in PD

1. http://www.everydayhealth.com/health-report/major-depression/
    depression-statistics.aspx
2. http://www.brainyquote.com/quotes/authors/m/marilyn_vos_savant.html
3. Chaudhuri RK, Prieto-Jurcynska C, Naidu Y, et al (2010): "The
    nondeclaration of nonmotor symptoms of Parkinson's disease to
    healthcare professionals. An international study using nonmotor
    questionnaire." Mov Disord 25(6):704-709.

4. http://anthropology.msu.edu/anp204-us12/2012/07/13/parkinsons-disease-among-hispanics-and-whites/

5. http://www.sciencedaily.com/releases/2010/01/100127164022.htm

6. http://www.alphagalileo.org/ViewItem.aspx?ItemId=139935&CultureCode=en

Chapter 18: Art Therapy: An Alternative Therapy for Treatment of PD

1. Gordon D. (December 2014): "Neurology then and now: How our understanding of five common neurological conditions has changed in 30years." Neurology Now; 33-35.

2. Biller K and Sussman M. (summer 2013): "Perception." US T.V series season 2, episode?

3. "Some Parkinson's Patients Discover an Artistic Side." (June 201). http://www.webmd.com/parkinsons-disease/news/20130131/some-parkinsons-patients-discover-an-artistic-side

4. American Friends of Tel Aviv University. "Parkinson's Treatment Can Trigger Creativity: Patients Treated with Dopamine-Enhancing Drugs are Developing Artistic Talents, Doctors Says." Science Daily. 14 January 2013. http://www.sciencedaily.com/releases/2013/01/130114111622.html

5. Ibid.

6. Pollak, T.A. "De Novo Artistic Behavior Following Brain Injury." http://www.ncbi.nlm.nrh.gov/pubmed1749506. 2007. Aug. 2013

7. Fung, Brian. "Eureka! When a Blow to the Head Creates a Sudden Genius." http://www.theatlantic.com/. . . /eureka-when-a-blow-to-the-head-creates-a. . . . may 172012

8. Ibid.

9. Schrag, A. and Trimble M. (March 2001): "Poetic talent unmasked by treatment of PD." Movement Disorder Journal 16 (6): 1175-1176.

10. Canesi M. Rusconi ML Isaias IU and Pelozzi G. (March 2012): "Artistic productivity and creativity in Parkinson's." European Journal of Neurology 19 (3):468-472.

11. Robynne, Boyd. "Do People Only Use 10 Percent of their Brains?: What's the Matter with Only Exploiting a Portion of Our Gray Matter?" http://www.scientificamerican.com/article-cfm?id=people-only-use-10 Sept.2013

12. Biller K and Sussman M. (summer 2014): "Perception" July 29, 2014.

13. Bogousslavsky J, Hennerici MG, Basel K. (Oct 2013): "Neurological Disorders in Famous Artists." http://books.google.com/books?ibbn=3805582655

14. Illness of Vincent Van Gogh: American Journal of psychiatry 159(4): 519. http://ajp.psychiatryonline.org/doi/full/10.1176/appi.ajp.159.4.519

15. http://en.m.wikipedia.org/wiki/Creativity_and_mental_illness

16. "Dopamine and the biology of creativity: lessons from Parkinson's disease." http://journal.frontiersin.org/Journal/10.3389/fneur.2014.00055/full

17. Bagan, B. "Expressive Arts. Aging, Alzheimer's, and Parkinson's: A manual for artists, art educators, health professionals, and others who work with older adults." 2009 Pg 8

18. Ibid.

19. Ibid pg9

20. Ibid pg8

21. Ibid pg 9

22. "Exploring the neural correlates of visual creativity" http://scan.oxfordjournals.org/content/early/2012/03/09/scan.nss021.full

23. Farrelly-Hansen, Mimi. "Spirituality & Art Therapy: living the Connection." Philadelphia. Jessica Kingsley Publishers 2003.

24. Bagan, B. "Expressive Arts. Aging, Alzheimer's, and Parkinson's: A manual for artists, art educators, health professionals, and others who work with older adults." 2009 Pg.8

25. Collier, AK (Dec 2014): "An app to spur creative expression in Alzheimer's patients." Neurology Now 23.

26. Canning L. (March 2004):"Are we more or less creative as we age?" Entrepreneur the Arts http://blog.entrepreneurthearts.com/2009/03/04/are-we-more-or-less-creative-as-we-age/

27. Ibid

28. Print awarenesshttp://en.m.wikipedia.org/wiki/Print_awareness

29. Faust-Socher A. et al (Jun 2014): "Enhanced creative thinking under dopaminergic therapy in Parkinson disease." Annals of Neurology http://onlinelibrary.wiley.com/doi/10.1002/ana.24181/abstract

30. "Two lives lost, a third forever changed." http://wwww.seattletimes.com/html/localnews/2010872336_lonimundell24m.html

31. (www.sharethecare.org/pages/share_advice/ALS_Peggychun.html;

32. www.islandartcards.com/shop/Artists_Showcase_Peggy_Chun_Prints.html

33. http://www.brainyquote.com/quotes/quotes/f/fscottfit 166303.html Aug 2013.

Chapter 19: Current Treatments: The Good, the Bad & the Promised Land

1. "Higher rates of certain cancers among LRRK2 gene Mutation carriers with PD." (Dec 2014): Science News. http://www.pdf.org/en/science_news/release/pr_1418740778

2. Kareus S, Figueroa KP, Cannon-Albright LA et. al. (Dec 2012): "Shared predispositions of Parkinsonism and cancer: A population-based pedigree-linked study." JAMA Neurology 69(12):1572-1577. Doi:10.1001/arcneurol.2012.2261.

3. http://www.rxlist.com/apokyn-side-effects-drug-center.htm

4. Marsh L and Callahan P. "Gambling, sex, and…Parkinson's disease?" Parkinson's Disease Foundation Newsletter. http://www.pdf.org/en/spring05_Gambling_Sex

5. Ibid.

6. "Naltrexone for impulse control disorders in Parkinsons disease/the Micheal J. Fox Foundation." https://www.michaeljfox.org/foundation/grant-detail.php?grant_id=567

7. "Deep brain stimulation effective in early Parkinson's." (Feb 2013): Science News http://www.pdf.org/en/science_news/release/pr_1361475315

8. Noonan D. (May 2014): "Inside the science of an amazing New surgery called deep brain stimulation: the most futuristic medical treatment ever imagined is now a reality." Smithsonian Magazine http://www.smithsonianmag.com/innovation/inside-science-amazing-new-surgery-called-deep-brain-stimulation-180951170/

9. "Parkinson's and Suicide." (Oct 2013) http://www.theparkinsonhub.com/your-quality-of-life/article/parkinsons-suicide.html

10. Yasgur BS. "Depression in Neurological disease." MPR. http://www.empr.com/depression-in-neurological-disease/article/283884/

11. Robin Williams: is Parkinson's disease linked to suicide? (Aug 2014): LiveScience. https://www.yahoo.com/health/robin-williams-is-parkinsons-disease-linked-to-94811585047.html

12. Ibid.

13. Voon V, Krack P, Lang AE et al. "A multicenter study on suicide outcomes following subthalamic stimulation for Parkinson's disease." (Oct. 2008)

Kullman DM. editor. Brain. A J of Neurology. http://doi.org/10.1093/brain/awn214 2720-2728.

14. Shah, Binit, B. "Focused Ultrasound For Parkinson's Tremor: An Update." Practical Neurology, November/December 23 2013, pg 19-20)

15. "New drug extends levodopa's benefits in moderate and advance Parkinson's disease." (Aug 2006) Science News. http://www.pdf.org/en/science_news/release/pr_1407337528

16. Chao OY, Mattern C, Silva AM, Wessler J. et. al. (Feb 2012): "Intranasally applied L-dopa alleviates parkinsonian symptoms in rats with unilateral nigro-striatal 6-OHDA lesions." BrainRes Bull 87(2-3):340-345. Doi. 10.1016/j.brainresbull.2011.11.004.Epub 2011 Nov 15.

17. "Duodopa intestinal gel-summary of product characteristics (SPC) – (eMC)." https://www.medicines.org.uk/emc/medicine/20786

18. Rajan C. (Sep 2014): "Acadia's Nuplazid receives FDA breakthrough therapy designation for Parkinson's psychosis." News Feature. http://www.bioprocessonline.com/doc/acadia-s-nuplazid-receives-fda-breakthrough-therapy-designation-for-parkinson-s-psychosis-0001

19. McGuire M. (March 2014): "Podcast: drug that May slow Parkinson's progression granted 423million from NIH for phase III testing." FoxFEED Blog https://www.michaeljfox.org/foundation/news-detail.php?podcast-drug-that-may-slow-parkinson-progression-granted-23-million-from-nih-for-phase-iii

20. Johnson H. (Dec 2014): "Parkinson's Disease Vaccine tested on First patients." http://www.business2community.com/health-wellness/parkinsons-disease-vaccine-tested-first-patients-01093546#HGmZoEXjCpg5A2FE.01

21. Olanow CW, Brundin P. (Jan 2013): "Parkinson's disease and alpha synuclein: is Parkinson's disease a prion-like disorder?" Mov Disord 28(1):31-40. Doi.10.1002/mds.25373.

Chapter 20: Nutrition Matters in PD

1. Susman E. (June 2013): "Curing H. pylori cuts Parkinson's symptoms."MedPage Today http://www.medpagetoday.com/MeetingCoverage/MDS/39967

2. Holden K. "Parkinson's Disease: nutrition matters." National Parkinson Foundation. Pg. 20

3. Columbia University Medical Center. "Is Parkinson's an autoimmune disease?" ScienceDaily. ScienceDaily. 17April 2014. http://www.sciencedaily.com/releases/2014/04/140417151227.htm

4. Jenkins B. (Feb 2011): "why your brain loves chocolate." http://www.scilearn.com/blog/why-your-brain-loves-chocolate

5. Sokolov AN, Pavlova MA, Klosterhalfen S, and Enck P. (Dec 2013): "Chocolate and the brain:neurobiological impact of cocoa flavanols on cognition and behavior." Neurosci Biobehav Rev. 37(10pt 2):2445-2453. Doi:10.1016/j.neubiorev.2013.06.013. Epub Jun 26.

6. Wolz M, Kaminsky A, Loehle M, et. al. (March 2009): "Chocolate consumption is increased in PD." 256(3):488-492.

7. Devgan L. (Aug 2013): "Is chocolate the new brain food?" http://abcnews.go.com/Health/ischocolate-the-new-brainfood/blogEntry?id=19901143&ref=https%3A%2F%2Fwww.google.com%2F

8. https://www.dosomething.org/facts/11-facts-about-chocolate

9. https://www.dosomething.org/facts/11-facts-about-chocolate

10. Jenkins B. (Feb 2011): "why your brain loves chocolate." http://www.scilearn.com/blog/why-your-brain-loves-chocolate

11. Rothschild, J. "5 Reasons Your Brain loves Chocolate." http://www.jenniferrothschild.com/5-reasons-your-brain-loves-chocolate/

12. Jenkins B. (Feb 2011): "why your brain loves chocolate." http://www.scilearn.com/blog/why-your-brain-loves-chocolate

1. Chapter 21: Caregiving in Parkinson's

1. Imke, Susan, RN, MS; Hutton, Tudy, JD; Loftus, Susan, RN, MSN. "National Parkinson's Foundation - Parkinson's Disease: Caring and Coping Brochure." Pg. 13

2. Ibid.

3. Ibid. pg 14.

4. Cooper A. (March 2010):"Depression and Resilience." Neurology Now 6(2):18-25.

5. Imke, Susan, RN, MS; Hutton, Tudy, JD; Loftus, Susan, RN, MSN. "National Parkinson's Foundation - Parkinson's Disease: Caring and Coping Brochure."

6. "A cup of Joe May help Some Parkinson's Disease symptoms." https://www.aan.com/pressroom/home/pressrelease/1096

7. (http://doc.mediaplanet.com/all projects/11984.pdf

8. Imke, Susan, RN, MS; Hutton, Tudy, JD; Loftus, Susan, RN, MSN. "National Parkinson's Foundation - Parkinson's Disease: Caring and Coping Brochure." Pg. 12

9. Angelou, Maya. "Continue." http://thesociologist.tumblr.com/
    post/87123774633/my-wish-for-you-is-that-you-continue-continue-to

Chapter 22: Wrap-up

1. Doty,R.Olfactory dysfunction in PD;Gaig C and Tolossa E When does
    PD begin?

2. "Higher rates of certain cancers among LRRK2 gene Mutation carriers
    with PD." (Dec 2014): Science News. http://www.pdf.org/en/science_
    news/release/pr_1418740778

3. Marras C. and Saunders-Pullman R. (June 2014) "Complexities of
    hormonal influences and risk of PD" Mov Disord 29 (7):845-848

4. "BRCA1 and BRCA2: Cancer Risk and Genetic testing." http://www.
    cancer.gov/cancertopics/factsheet/Risk/BRCA

5. http://wwwsciencedaily.com/release/2014/04/140417151227.htm).

6. Menstruation and menopause: EPDA: http://www.epda.eu.com/en/
    parkinsons/in-depth/managing-your-parkinsons/daily-living/women-
    parkinsons/menstruation-menopause/

7. Liu R., Baird Donna, Park Yikyung et al. (June 2014) "Female
    reproductive factors, menopausal hormone use, and Parkinson's disease."
    Mov disord 29 (7):889-896

8. Plotkin G. Director of the Movement Disorder Clinic at ETMC of
    Neurological Institute at ETMC

9. Science News (Nov 2014): study finds that mental health issues lead
    people with Parkinson's to leave the workforce." PDF http://www.pdf.org/
    en/ science_news/release/pr_1415296989

10. Science News (Nov 2014): study finds that mental health issues lead
    people with Parkinson's to leave the workforce." PDF http://www.pdf.org/
    en/ science_news/release/pr_1415296989

11. Wayant, Patricia editor. (2012) Words Every Woman Should Remember:
    Messages of support, Encouragement, and Gratitude for all you are and all
    you do. Blue Mountain Press. Page.39

12. http://www.brainyquote.com/quotes/quotes/a/audreyhepb126745.html

13. Wayant, Patricia editor. (2012) Words Every Woman Should Remember:
    Messages of support, Encouragement, and Gratitude for all you are and all
    you do. Blue Mountain Press. Page.28

14. Markman, Art (May 2010): "Say it Loud: I'm creating a distinctive
    memory." Psychology Today. https://www.psychologytoday.com/blog/
    ulterior-motives/201005/say-it-loud-i-m-creating-distinctive-memory

15. Orman Suze. (2007) Women and Money: Owning the power to control your destiny page 246-247.

CPSIA information can be obtained
at www.ICGtesting.com
Printed in the USA
BVHW08s0535130818
524258BV00002B/44/P